T0226615

Pregnancy and Neurologic Illness

Guest Editor

AUTUMN KLEIN, MD, PhD

NEUROLOGIC CLINICS

www.neurologic.theclinics.com

Consulting Editor
RANDOLPH W. EVANS, MD

August 2012 • Volume 30 • Number 3

SAUNDERS an imprint of ELSEVIER, Inc.

W.B. SAUNDERS COMPANY
A Division of Elsevier Inc.

1600 John F. Kennedy Boulevard • Suite 1800 • Philadelphia, Pennsylvania 19103-2899

http://www.theclinics.com

NEUROLOGIC CLINICS Volume 30, Number 3
August 2012 ISSN 0733-8619, ISBN-13: 978-1-4557-3895-3

Editor: Donald Mumford

Neurologic Clinics (ISSN 0733-8619) is published quarterly by Elsevier Inc., 360 Park Avenue South, New York, NY 10010–1710. Months of issue are February, May, August, and November. Periodicals postage paid at New York, NY, and additional mailing offices. Subscription prices are $285.00 per year for US individuals, $470.00 per year for US institutions, $140.00 per year for US students, $359.00 per year for Canadian individuals, $564.00 per year for Canadian institutions, $397.00 per year for international individuals, $564.00 per year for international institutions, and $199.00 for Canadian and foreign students/residents. To receive student/resident rate, orders must be accompanied by name of affiliated institution, date of term, and the *signature* of program/residency coordinator on institution letterhead. Orders will be billed at individual rate until proof of status is received. Foreign air speed delivery is included in all *Clinics* subscription prices. All prices are subject to change without notice. **POSTMASTER:** Send address changes to *Neurologic Clinics*, Elsevier Health Sciences Division, Subscription Customer Service, 3251 Riverport Lane, Maryland Heights, MO 63043. **Customer Service: Telephone: 1-800-654-2452 (U.S. and Canada); 314-447-8871 (outside U.S. and Canada). Fax: 314-447-8029. E-mail: journalscustomerservice-usa@elsevier.com (for print support); journalsonlinesupport-usa@elsevier.com (for online support).**

Reprints. For copies of 100 or more of articles in this publication, please contact the Commercial Reprints Department, Elsevier Inc., 360 Park Avenue South, New York, New York, 10010-1710; Tel.: (+1) 212-633-3812; Fax: (+1) 212-462-1935, and E-mail: reprints@elsevier.com.

Neurologic Clinics is also published in Spanish by Nueva Editorial Interamericana S.A., Mexico City, Mexico.

Neurologic Clinics is covered in *Current Contents/Clinical Medicine, MEDLINE/PubMed (Index Medicus), EMBASE/Excerpta Medica, and PsycINFO, and ISI/BIOMED.*

Printed and bound by CPI Group (UK) Ltd, Croydon, CR0 4YY
Transferred to Digital Print 2012

Contributors

CONSULTING EDITOR

RANDOLPH W. EVANS, MD
Clinical Professor, Department of Neurology, Baylor College of Medicine, Houston, Texas

GUEST EDITOR

AUTUMN KLEIN, MD, PhD
Chief, Division of Women's Neurology; Assistant Professor of Neurology and Obstetrics and Gynecology, Department of Neurology, UPMC Presbyterian/Magee Womens Hospital of UPMC, University of Pittsburgh, Pittsburgh, Pennsylvania

AUTHORS

CHRISTOPHER M. BONFIELD, MD
Department of Neurological Surgery, University of Pittsburgh Medical Center, Pittsburgh, Pennsylvania

JUSTINE CHANG, MD
Fellow, Division of Maternal-Fetal Medicine, Department of Obstetrics, Gynecology, and Reproductive Sciences, Magee-Womens Hospital, University of Pittsburgh, Pittsburgh, Pennsylvania

P.K. COYLE, MD
Professor of Neurology, Director, Department of Neurology, Stony Brook MS Comprehensive Care Center, Stony Brook University, Stony Brook, New York

WILLIAM T. DELFYETT, MD
Assistant Professor of Neuroradiology, Department of Radiology, UPMC Presbyterian Hospital, University of Pittsburgh School of Medicine, UPMC Presbyterian-Shadyside, Pittsburgh, Pennsylvania

JOHNATHAN A. ENGH, MD
Department of Neurological Surgery, University of Pittsburgh Medical Center, Pittsburgh, Pennsylvania

DAVID T. FETZER, MD
Diagnostic Radiology Resident, PGY-V, UPMC Medical Graduate Program, University of Pittsburgh School of Medicine; Department of Radiology, Radiology Residency Program at UPMC, Pittsburgh, Pennsylvania

NANCY FOLDVARY-SCHAEFER, DO, MS
Director, Associate Professor of Neurology, Cleveland Clinic Lerner College of Medicine, Cleveland Clinic Sleep Disorders Center, Cleveland, Ohio

AMANDA C. GUIDON, MD
Division of Neurology, Department of Medicine, Duke University Medical Center, Durham, North Carolina

SALLY IBRAHIM, MD
Staff, Cleveland Clinic Sleep Disorders Center, Neurological Institute, Cleveland, Ohio

AUTUMN KLEIN, MD, PhD
Chief, Division of Women's Neurology; Assistant Professor of Neurology and Obstetrics and Gynecology, Department of Neurology and Obstetrics and Gynecology, UPMC Presbyterian/Magee Womens Hospital of UPMC, Pittsburgh, Pennsylvania

OLAJIDE KOWE, MBBS, FCARCSI
Department of Anesthesiology, Magee-Womens Hospital of University of Pittsburgh Medical Center, Pittsburgh, Pennsylvania

E. ANNE MACGREGOR, MB BS, MD, MFSRH, MICR
Honorary Professor, Barts Sexual Health Centre, St Bartholomew's Hospital; Honorary Professor, Centre for Neuroscience and Trauma, Blizard Institute of Cell and Molecular Science, Barts and the London School of Medicine and Dentistry, London, United Kingdom

E. WAYNE MASSEY, MD
Division of Neurology, Department of Medicine, Duke University Medical Center, Durham, North Carolina

DAVID STREITMAN, MD
Assistant Professor, Division of Maternal-Fetal Medicine, Department of Obstetrics, Gynecology, and Reproductive Sciences, Magee-Womens Hospital, University of Pittsburgh, Pittsburgh, Pennsylvania

BARBARA TETTENBORN, MD, PhD
Professor of Neurology, Professor, University of Mainz, Mainz, Germany; University of Zürich, Zürich; Head of Department of Neurology, Kantonsspital St Gallen, St Gallen, Switzerland

JONATHAN H. WATERS, MD
Department of Anesthesiology, Magee-Womens Hospital of University of Pittsburgh Medical Center, Pittsburgh, Pennsylvania

Contents

Preface   ix

Autumn Klein

Physiologic Adaptations to Pregnancy   781

Justine Chang and David Streitman

> Pregnancy leads to diverse physiologic changes to accommodate the de-
> mands of the developing fetoplacental unit, which affect many major organ
> systems. Understanding these physiologic adaptations to pregnancy is
> important for all clinicians because they have important implications for
> the diagnosis and management of various disorders. This article provides
> a brief overview of the most notable of these adaptations, including cardio-
> vascular, hematologic, respiratory, renal, immunologic, and gastrointesti-
> nal. Clinical correlate of pharmacokinetics and a patient case study are
> included.

Imaging of Neurologic Conditions During Pregnancy and the Perinatal Period   791

William T. Delfyett and David T. Fetzer

> Throughout pregnancy and the puerperium, a variety of hormonal and
> physiologic changes occur that are associated with pregnancy-specific
> neurologic conditions, which may also influence known preexisting medi-
> cal conditions or bring previously unknown neurologic conditions to clini-
> cal attention. This article reviews the imaging of a spectrum of neurologic
> conditions that may be encountered in the pregnant or puerperal patient,
> the key physiologic changes that are most germane to the imaging of neu-
> rologic conditions, and the important safety considerations that are made
> when choosing and performing a diagnostic imaging test for the pregnant
> and puerperal patient.

Neurologic Complications in the Patient Receiving Obstetric Anesthesia   823

Olajide Kowe and Jonathan H. Waters

> Neurologic deficits during or following labor and delivery often occur as
> a result of obstetric trauma. They can also be caused by neuraxial (epidural
> or spinal) anesthesia. The incidence of obstetric anesthesia neuropathy is
> unknown. Anesthesia can cause neurologic injury, although the mecha-
> nisms for these injuries are different from those of obstetric injury. Injury
> can result from direct trauma to the spinal cord, epidural hematoma, as
> well as other causes that are discussed in this article. These injuries are
> less common than those of birth trauma.

Headache in Pregnancy   835

E. Anne MacGregor

> Primary headaches are most common in women during their reproductive
> years and are affected by the hormonal fluctuations during pregnancy.
> Most headaches follow a benign course during pregnancy, although mi-
> graine is associated with increased risk of hypertensive disorders of

pregnancy and stroke. Management of primary headaches during pregnancy is essentially similar to management in the nonpregnant state, with a few exceptions. This article reviews the epidemiology, prognosis, and management of primary headaches during pregnancy and lactation, and considers secondary headaches that are important to exclude.

The Postpartum Period in Women with Epilepsy   867

Autumn Klein

For women with epilepsy (WWE), the postpartum period is a vulnerable time owing to medication alterations, disrupted sleep, increased stress, and the challenges of breastfeeding. Sleep deprivation and the stress of having a new child can be challenging for WWE. Concerns over antiepileptic drugs (AEDs) in breast milk and sleep disruption associated with breastfeeding leads some WWE to discontinue breastfeeding. Adjustment of AEDs in the postpartum period can lead to difficulties in seizure control. Postpartum depression is increased in WWE, and patient education about newborn safety remains a concern. This article covers these important topics in postpartum WWE.

Pregnancy and Multiple Sclerosis   877

P.K. Coyle

Pregnancy is a major concern in multiple sclerosis (MS), because the typical patient is a young woman of childbearing age. This article reviews the impact of pregnancy on MS. Disease activity decreases, particularly during the last trimester. There is a temporary rebound of disease activity in the 3 months postpartum. Pregnancy and the postpartum period have many implications for counseling and for therapeutic decision making in MS.

Neuromuscular Disorders in Pregnancy   889

Amanda C. Guidon and E. Wayne Massey

Preexisting and coincident neuromuscular disorders in pregnancy are challenging for clinicians because of the heterogeneity of disease and the limited data in the literature. Many questions arise regarding the effect of disease on the pregnancy, delivery, and newborn in addition to the effect of pregnancy on the course of disease. Each disorder has particular considerations and possible complications. An interdisciplinary team of physicians is essential. This article discusses the most recent literature on neuromuscular disorders in pregnancy including acquired root, plexus, and peripheral nerve lesions; acquired and inherited neuropathies and myopathies; disorders of the neuromuscular junction; and motor neuron diseases.

Stroke and Pregnancy   913

Barbara Tettenborn

Strategies for stroke prevention should take into account the competing risks to mother and fetus. Treatment of acute stroke in pregnant women is still controversial, but not strictly contraindicated. Several case reports have documented successful reperfusion, in addition to satisfactory maternal and fetal outcomes. Aspirin and warfarin are safe in the second and third trimesters. There are no trials of anticoagulation or antiplatelet therapies of stroke prevention in pregnancy.

Sleep Disorders in Pregnancy: Implications, Evaluation, and Treatment   **925**

Sally Ibrahim and Nancy Foldvary-Schaefer

The dynamic changes across pregnancy affect sleep and wakefulness producing sleep disturbances, which causes sleep disorders in some cases. This review will identify common sleep disorders in pregnancy, related maternal-fetal outcomes, pathophysiologic mechanisms, and potential therapies to guide clinicians in serving this population.

Pregnancy and Brain Tumors   **937**

Christopher M. Bonfield and Johnathan A. Engh

This article discusses the clinical presentation, diagnosis, and treatment of the pregnant patient with an intracranial mass. Common manifestations, pitfalls, and guidelines for management are discussed.

Index   **947**

NEUROLOGIC CLINICS

FORTHCOMING ISSUES

November 2012
Sleep Disorders
Bradley W. Vaughn, MD, *Guest Editor*

February 2013
Spinal Cord Diseases and Disorders
Alireza Minagar, MD, FAAN, and
Alejandro A. Rabinstein, MD, FAAN,
Guest Editors

May 2013
Peripheral Neuropathy
Richard Barohn, MD, *Guest Editor*

RECENT ISSUES

May 2012
Clinical Electromyography
Devon I. Rubin, MD, *Guest Editor*

February 2012
Neurologic Emergencies
Alireza Minagar, MD, FAAN, and
Alejandro A. Rabinstein, MD, FAAN,
Guest Editors

November 2011
Disorders of Consciousness
G. Bryan Young, MD, *Guest Editor*

RELATED INTEREST

Clinics in Perinatology, December 2009, (Volume 36, Issue 4)
Neurology of the Newborn Infant
Adré J. du Plessis, MBChB, MPH, *Guest Editor*

DOWNLOAD
Free App!

Review Articles
THE CLINICS

NOW AVAILABLE FOR YOUR iPhone and iPad

Preface

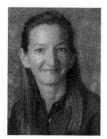

Autumn Klein, MD, PhD
Guest Editor

Many neurologists have little experience with evaluating, diagnosing, and managing a pregnant woman, yet in a large general neurology practice or at an academic center, it is not uncommon to see several pregnant women a month. Many physicians think of a pregnant woman as a patient who cannot get certain tests and who generally cannot take medications. What many physicians may not appreciate is that the physiology of pregnancy leads to changes in neurological disease presentation that may not be typical in the nonpregnant state. In addition, neurological diseases follow specific patterns during pregnancy that, if known, can provide guidance and reassurance. The articles in this issue of *Neurologic Clinics* hope to enlighten neurologists about situations with which they are unfamiliar and likely need more education. Cases have been included to highlight practical challenges.

Optimal care for the obstetrical patient with a neurological issue requires an interdisciplinary team. The authorship of these articles reflects this. The first few articles provide input from outside neurology in related specialties including obstetrics, radiology, and anesthesia. The following articles are written by a group of expert subspecialists in neurology who have a particular interest in neurological issues in pregnancy and have experience seeing pregnant patients.

The issue begins with a neurologist's version of basic obstetrical physiology. This article reminds neurologists of the changes in the pregnant body, such as hypercoagulable factors, that may influence neurological disease. The next article on neuroradiology will review the basic concepts involved in imaging a pregnant woman, such as radiation exposure, and the risks associated with iodinated contrast and gadolinium. A unique contribution comes from obstetrical anesthesia. Many neurologists do not appreciate the different anesthetic techniques that pregnant women may undergo, and this article helps to outline the forethought, the detailed techniques, and the risks and concerns of these procedures (epidural, spinal, intubation) in pregnant women.

Next are the subspecialties in neurology and the issues uniquely encountered by each of them. Headache, epilepsy, peripheral neuropathy, and multiple sclerosis are the most common neurological issues in pregnancy, and each of these articles highlights the key points encountered in these diseases. Stroke, albeit uncommon in pregnancy, is devastating when it happens to young people and is a major concern when

Neurol Clin 30 (2012) ix–x
http://dx.doi.org/10.1016/j.ncl.2012.06.005
0733-8619/12/$ – see front matter © 2012 Elsevier Inc. All rights reserved.

neurologic.theclinics.com

someone presents with neurological deficits in pregnancy. While sleep disorders in pregnancy may seem obvious (frequent arousals due to urinating at night and discomfort in sleep), sleep in pregnancy is more complex, and there is still much to understand about it. Finally, in the spirit of an interdisciplinary topic, neurosurgical issues in pregnancy have been included. Many neurologists may be consulted on these patients who have both neurological and neurosurgical issues (ie, headache and shunt) and, again, it is an area with which many neurologists are unfamiliar.

I would like to send out a special thanks to Donald Mumford, who was instrumental in helping me pull this together. His patience and persistence made this publication possible. I also want to thank all of the authors who contributed to this issue of *Neurologic Clinics*. Their collective expertise is impressive, and my hope is that the readers will benefit from their education and insight as much as I have.

Autumn Klein, MD, PhD
Division of Women's Neurology
Department of Neurology and Obstetrics and Gynecology
UPMC Presbyterian/Magee Womens Hospital of UPMC
University of Pittsburgh
Kaufmann Medical Building
3471 Fifth Avenue, Suite 811
Pittsburgh, PA 15213, USA

E-mail address:
kleinam2@upmc.edu

Physiologic Adaptations to Pregnancy

Justine Chang, MD, David Streitman, MD*

KEYWORDS

- Pregnancy • Physiology • Adaptation

KEY POINTS

- Cardiovascular adaptation to pregnancy begins early, continues steadily from late first trimester to term, and rapid shifts occur postpartum. These alterations in physiology can have profound effect on disease processes unrelated to pregnancy.
- Vascular and tissue congestion in the upper airway, along with increased aspiration risk mechanisms, can lead to difficult airway management during seizure or other severe neurologic compromise.
- Renal function enhancements parallel cardiovascular changes across pregnancy and often lead to altered drug metabolism and clearance. Along with increases in serum drug binding proteins and metabolic enzymes, renal adaptation to pregnancy should prompt consideration of medication dosage adjustment.
- Gastrointestinal changes can shift from inability to ingest medications or adequate nutrients and fluids, to more frequent ingestion of nutrients that may bind medications and alter bioavailability, to slowed gastrointestinal motility with altered absorption of scheduled medications. These changes should be considered when tailoring medication dosages and when counseling patients about medication regimens.

INTRODUCTION

Pregnancy induces significant maternal physiologic changes to accommodate the demands of the developing fetoplacental unit. The following discussion is meant to serve as a brief overview of the most notable of these physiologic adaptations.

CARDIOVASCULAR CHANGES

Beginning in the first trimester, the cardiovascular system demonstrates changes that optimize oxygen and nutrient delivery to the growing fetus. Cardiac output has been

The authors have nothing to disclose.
Division of Maternal-Fetal Medicine, Department of Obstetrics, Gynecology, and Reproductive Sciences, Magee-Womens Hospital, University of Pittsburgh, 300 Halket Street, Pittsburgh, PA 15213, USA
* Corresponding author.
E-mail address: streitmandc@mail.magee.edu

Neurol Clin 30 (2012) 781–789
doi:10.1016/j.ncl.2012.05.001
0733-8619/12/$ – see front matter © 2012 Elsevier Inc. All rights reserved.

neurologic.theclinics.com

noted to increase from the early first trimester[1]; cardiac output increases progressively and reaches its peak values, which are on average 30% to 50% more than preconception levels by 25- to 30-weeks gestation (an increase from 4 L/minute to 6 L/minute).[2] This dramatic increase in cardiac output is even more pronounced in multifetal gestation; peak cardiac output in twin gestations is 20% higher than in singleton pregnancies.[3] This increase in cardiac output reflects an increase in stroke volume as well as heart rate.[4] The increase in maternal heart rate seems to plateau in the third trimester with average rates 15 to 20 beats per minute more than the baseline nonpregnant heart rate. Stroke volume also increases by approximately 40% during the course of gestation.[5,6]

This increased cardiac output is redistributed in pregnancy to favor perfusion to the uterus and placenta, kidneys, breasts, and skin. In pregnancy, by term, blood flow to the uteroplacental unit comprises 20% to 25% of maternal cardiac output (approximately 500 mL/minute) and renal blood flow represents 20% of maternal cardiac output.[5] The skin and breasts receive 10% and 2% of maternal cardiac output, respectively. The increase in blood flow to the skin may be adaptive in that it allows dissipation of heat generated by fetal metabolism.

Although decreased cerebral blood flow has been observed during pregnancy (specifically, decreased middle cerebral artery blood flow has been observed with transcranial Doppler sonography of healthy pregnant women[7]), there is no apparent change in cerebral autoregulation during pregnancy.[8] The maintenance of cerebral autoregulation in pregnancy is also demonstrated in studies that show no change in middle cerebral artery blood flow with regional anesthesia that is associated with significant changes in maternal hemodynamic parameters.[9]

In the second and third trimesters, cardiac output is sensitive to maternal position. In the dorsal supine position, the gravid uterus may compress the inferior vena cava leading to impaired venous blood return to the heart. This decrease in preload can result in a significant drop in cardiac output (10%–30% decrease) that may lead to symptomatic maternal hypotension (can affect cerebral perfusion; creates presyncope and nausea) as well as to decreased perfusion of the uterus and placenta resulting in fetal compromise.[10] If women in the second or third trimesters undergo procedures (eg, head or neck imaging) that require supine positioning, modifying the position to the left lateral decubitus is recommended (this is accomplished with the placement of a wedge under the right hip).

Reversible myocardial hypertrophy is also noted during pregnancy; this likely occurs in response to the expanded blood volume of pregnancy. The cardiac chambers also enlarge, with atrial diameters 40% larger than their prepregnant values.[11] The dilatation of the atria in conjunction with the increased heart rate in pregnancy and changes in hormones such as estrogen may all contribute to a greater risk of arrhythmias. In observational studies, the most common arrhythmias noted were benign premature atrial or ventricular contractions.[12,13]

Blood pressures in pregnancy tend to be lower than nonpregnant values. Systemic vascular resistance declines with a nadir in the second trimester (at around 20-weeks gestation) followed by a gradual increase until term. At term, the systemic vascular resistance is still approximately 20% lower than what is observed prepregnancy.[14,15] The underlying mechanism of this decrease in systemic vascular resistance is unclear but is likely multifactorial. Progesterone likely exerts some effects on vascular smooth muscle relaxation and increases in nitric oxide in pregnancy likely contribute to changes in vascular resistance.[16]

The cardiovascular changes of pregnancy may alter physical examination findings and be mistaken for evidence of cardiac disease. In the second and third trimesters, peripheral edema is a common finding as is lateral displacement of the apex of the left ventricle. Jugular venous distention may also be noted in late gestation without underlying cardiac pathologic condition. Systolic ejection murmurs auscultated over the left sternal border are also common findings and are attributed to increased blood flow across the aortic valve. Many women will also demonstrate a third heart sound (S3) later in pregnancy related to rapid diastolic filling of the left ventricle that is common in the third trimester.[17]

Intrapartum, increased cardiac output results from elevated autonomic output related to pain from contractions (leading to elevated heart rate and arterial blood pressures) as well as from the contractions themselves (autotransfusion of approximately 300–500 mL blood increases venous return to the heart during each contraction). Mean arterial pressure also increases in parallel with the changes in cardiac output intrapartum.[18–21] The degree of change in cardiac output is affected by maternal position as well as regional analgesia.[22] Changes in cardiac output are more pronounced with patients in the lateral recumbent position as compared with the supine position. Regional analgesia blunts the increase in cardiac output, likely due to increased venous capacitance. Maximum cardiac output occurs immediately postpartum (within 10–30 minutes after delivery) and is possibly related to uterine autotransfusion that occurs following delivery of the fetus and placenta. The cardiovascular alterations related to pregnancy resolve during the first 4 to 12 postpartum weeks.[1]

HEMATOLOGIC CHANGES

The hematologic system also undergoes dramatic changes in response to pregnancy. Expansion of both plasma and red blood cell volumes leads to an expansion of total blood volume by approximately 1500 to 1600 mL. The expansion in plasma volume has been noted to begin in the first trimester and seems to plateau by 32- to 34-weeks gestation. During the course of pregnancy, the plasma volume increases by approximately 1200 to 1300 mL, which represents an approximately 40% increase in volume compared with nonpregnant women. Red blood cell mass increases by approximately 18% to 25% during the course of pregnancy.[23–25] Because the plasma volume increases more significantly than red blood cell volume, most pregnant women develop a "physiologic anemia." Iron deficiency during pregnancy is also frequent because appropriate development of the fetal hematologic system requires increased maternal iron stores; the overall iron requirements in pregnancy are estimated to be 1000 mg.[26]

Pregnancy represents a prothrombotic state. The risk of venous thromboembolism is four times greater in pregnancy and, especially, the postpartum period compared with the nonpregnant state.[27,28] Procoagulant factors (I, VII, VIII, IX, and X), as well as fibrinogen, are produced in greater quantities during pregnancy.[29] Meanwhile, factors important in fibrinolysis (eg, plasminogen activator) seem to be decreased in pregnancy. Additionally, impaired venous return from the lower extremities due to compression of the pelvic veins and inferior vena cava contribute to increased venous stasis, which also further increases the risk of thrombus formation.[30]

RESPIRATORY CHANGES

During pregnancy, the ligaments between the ribs and the sternum become more lax, allowing for an increase in the diameter of the thorax by 2 cm or more; the level of the diaphragm elevates 4 cm over the course of gestation.[31] These changes contribute to an overall decrease in total lung capacity by approximately 5%, and functional residual capacity (the volume of air in the lungs at the end of normal expiration) decreases by approximately 20%. Hyperventilation in pregnancy is also noted in response to an increase in tidal volume by approximately 30% to 50% despite a normal respiratory rate. This facilitates an increase in gas exchange with an increased alveolar partial pressure of oxygen and a decreased partial pressure of arterial carbon dioxide. Pregnancy is a state of respiratory alkalosis that facilitates improved carbon dioxide transfer from the fetal to the maternal circulation. The kidneys compensate for this chronic respiratory alkalosis (mean arterial pH around 7.43) by increasing excretion of bicarbonate (resulting in mean serum levels of bicarbonate of 21.5 mmol/L).[32–35]

Maternal oxygen consumption increases over gestation reflecting the increasing demands of the growing fetus and placenta. The combination of increased oxygen consumption and decreased functional residual capacity results in an overall decreased maternal oxygen reserve. Pregnant women, therefore, have a greater risk of complications when faced with respiratory compromise (eg, apnea in the setting of seizures, pneumonia, or asthma exacerbation).

Intubation in pregnancy should only be performed by experienced providers because maternal changes in the respiratory and gastrointestinal tract cause an increased risk of complications with this procedure. In pregnancy, the mucosa of the upper airway (nasopharynx) becomes hyperemic and edematous with increased mucus production.

Elevated progesterone levels in pregnancy appear to decrease gastrointestinal motility and lead to relaxation of the gastroesophageal sphincter; these changes as well as increased intraabdominal pressure from the gravid uterus all make emesis and aspiration a greater risk with sedation and intubation in pregnancy.[36,37] The complications associated with the greatest risks of maternal morbidity and mortality are difficulty achieving adequate intubation, esophageal intubation, and difficult or traumatic intubation.[38,39] In pregnancy, rates of difficult or failed intubation exceed those seen in non-pregnant women; in one observational series, 3.3% of women were felt to have had a difficult intubation while 0.3% had a failed intubation.[40]

RENAL CHANGES

Renal blood flow is increased from the first trimester of pregnancy, with an increase of approximately 50% across gestation when compared with nonpregnant levels. The glomerular filtration rate also increases significantly over the course of gestation to rates 50% higher than in the nonpregnant state. This results in a reduction in serum creatinine and urea concentrations with average concentrations in pregnancy of 0.5 mg/dL and 9.0 mg/dL, respectively. A decrease in renal vascular resistance likely contributes to the increase in renal blood flow. This decrease in resistance is likely mediated by pregnancy hormones (eg, progesterone and relaxin), although the underlying mechanisms have not been fully elucidated.[41–43] Alterations in renal filtration produce the increase in total body water that is necessary for providing adequate water content for the fetus and placenta, as well as facilitating the expansion in blood volume previously described. Sodium and water retention result from increased activity of the renin-angiotensin-aldosterone system during pregnancy.[44,45]

IMMUNOLOGIC CHANGES

Immunologic adaptations that occur in pregnancy likely arise to ensure maternal tolerance of the semiallogeneic fetus. Studies evaluating changes in immune cell populations and function indicate a possible decreased cytotoxic immune response with preservation of humoral and innate immunity. Pregnancy-related changes in hormones such as progesterone, estrogen, and relaxin may mediate changes in immune cell function and cytokine production. For example, both progesterone and estrogen have been shown to promote production of the antiinflammatory cytokine IL-10, which downregulates cytokines important in the cell-mediated cytotoxic immune response.[46,47] These changes in the maternal immune system may explain the observation that certain autoimmune disorders with a significant cell-mediated component (eg, multiple sclerosis and rheumatoid arthritis) seem to improve during pregnancy.[48]

GASTROINTESTINAL CHANGES

Nausea and vomiting of pregnancy are commonly encountered complaints affecting 70% to 85% of pregnant women, usually in the first trimester. Although the underlying mechanism is not clear, it seems that pregnancy-specific hormones such as human chorionic gonadotropin (hCG) play a role in mediating these symptoms. hCG peaks in the first trimester and begins to decrease in concentration by the beginning of the second trimester, by which point most women experience improvement in their symptoms. Twin gestations are associated with higher levels of hCG and a greater risk for nausea and vomiting related to pregnancy.[49] Pregnancy is associated with an increased incidence of reflux esophagitis due to the decreased gastrointestinal motility and decreased gastroesophageal sphincter tone, which likely result from the actions of progesterone.

DRUG METABOLISM CHANGES

Many of the physiologic changes of pregnancy may alter the pharmacokinetics of various drugs. Increases in total body water may increase the volume of distribution of drugs. Decreases in total protein and albumin concentrations may occur as a result of hemodilution, which may also change protein binding of certain medications, thus altering their peak concentrations leading to increasing free levels of these drugs over the course of gestation. Increased glomerular filtration may also increase the rate of clearance of renally eliminated medications.[50] Hepatic drug metabolizing enzymes may be influenced by hormonal changes. Studies have demonstrated a change in cytochrome P450 (CYP) enzyme activity levels during pregnancy. For example, CYP3A4 activity was significantly increased in pregnancy, whereas CYP1A2 activity was significantly decreased throughout gestation.[51] *Additionally, the placenta may also have drug transporting or metabolizing mechanisms that further alter drug levels during pregnancy. Delays in gastrointestinal transit time and increases in gastric pH during pregnancy may alter drug absorption, though the overall impact on bioavailability of these changes has not been well defined in many instances.[52,53]* Nausea and vomiting associated with pregnancy may also impair compliance with prescribed medications.

SUMMARY

Pregnancy leads to diverse physiologic changes that affect many major organ systems. Understanding these physiologic adaptations to pregnancy is important for all clinicians because they have important implications for the diagnosis and management of various disorders.

PATIENT CASE STUDY

A 19 year old G2P0010 at 38-weeks gestation presents complaining of persistent headache not responsive to Tylenol. She describes the headache as being diffuse but greatest in the occipital region and it has been unremitting for the past 24 hours; she has not previously experienced a headache like this. She denies any other complaints. She has no significant past medical history and her pregnancy had been uncomplicated before her presentation. During her evaluation, she was noted to have newly elevated blood pressure of 150s/90s. Her physical examination was notable only for brisk, symmetric patellar reflexes bilaterally. Laboratory analysis was notable for hemoglobin of 14 g/dL, a platelet count of 100,000, a creatinine of 1.0 mg/dL, and a urinalysis that demonstrated 3+ protein.

Important Points

- Recognition of abnormal blood pressure in pregnancy.
- Laboratory abnormalities: hemoglobin concentration is usually low due to physiologic anemia of pregnancy; in pre-eclampsia, vascular endothelial damage allows loss of serum osmotic factors to tissue interstitial space, causing hemoconcentration. Serum creatinine is usually low due to increased renal filtration rate; in pre-eclampsia, loss of plasma volume during hemoconcentration leads to elevated creatinine.

The patient was admitted to the labor and delivery unit with a diagnosis of preeclampsia. Given her term gestational age, the decision was made to proceed toward delivery with induction of labor. En route to the labor and delivery unit, the patient complained of sudden worsening of her headache and had a witnessed generalized tonic-clonic seizure lasting approximately 90 seconds. The patient was placed in the left lateral decubitus position; oxygen was administered by facemask and a 6 g intravenous bolus of magnesium was given followed by a maintenance infusion of 2 g per hour. During this time, the fetal heart rate tracing was notable for a prolonged deceleration to the 80s, but this resolved after 3 minutes in parallel with improvement in maternal respiration and oxygenation. A limited neurologic examination did not demonstrate any focal abnormalities but, given the patient's sudden worsening of headache before onset of seizure, the decision was made to proceed with head imaging to evaluate for a possible intracranial bleed before formulating a delivery plan. A noncontrast head CT scan was performed that was negative for any acute intracranial abnormalities.

Important Points

CT imaging, especially of the head and neck, is associated with low fetal radiation exposure (typically <1 radiation absorbed dose); radiation exposure at this dosage, especially later in gestation, has not been associated with increased risks of fetal malformation or pregnancy loss.

An induction of labor was initiated. During the course of her induction, the patient was noted to have increasing blood pressure to the 170s/110s. Given persistence of this severe degree of hypertension, the decision was made to administer antihypertensives in the form of intravenous labetalol. Soon after administration, the patient complained of severe nausea and lightheadedness and the fetal heart rate tracing was noted to demonstrate fetal bradycardia. The patient's blood pressure was noted to be 80/48.

Important Points

In preeclampsia, there is likely an element of endothelial dysfunction. This element, in conjunction with decreased colloid oncotic pressure from protein loss in the urine, can lead to decreased intravascular volume. In this setting, vasodilation from antihypertensive agents can lead to severe hypotension.

The patient was resuscitated with an intravenous fluid bolus to improve intravascular volume status, and with repositioning in the lateral position.

Important Points

Avoiding the supine position is important in this setting. The gravid uterus can compress the inferior vena cava, thus impairing venous return from the lower extremities and pelvis and limiting preload to the heart.

The patient ultimately required a cesarean delivery due to a failed induction of labor. Although an epidural had been placed, anesthesia sufficient for surgery was unable to be achieved so general endotracheal anesthesia was necessary. Two attempts at intubation were necessary but, ultimately, the patient was successfully intubated and underwent an uncomplicated cesarean delivery.

Important Points

Intubation in pregnancy is associated with increased risks of complications. Intubation may be technically more challenging owing to increased airway edema in pregnancy, which may be especially pronounced in women with preeclampsia. Aspiration risk is also elevated in pregnancy. Hypoxia may develop rapidly during attempts at intubation owing to decreased functional residual capacity observed during pregnancy.

REFERENCES

1. Capeless EL, Clapp JF. When do cardiovascular parameters return to their preconception values? Am J Obstet Gynecol 1991;165:883–6.
2. Bader RA, Bader ME, Jose DJ, et al. Hemodynamics at rest and during exercise in normal pregnancy as studied by cardiac catheterization. J Clin Invest 1955;34:1524–36.
3. Kametas NA, McAuliffe F, Krampl E, et al. Maternal cardiac function in twin pregnancy. Obstet Gynecol 2003;102:806–15.
4. Clark SL, Cotton DB, Lee W, et al. Central hemodynamic assessment of normal term pregnancy. Am J Obstet Gynecol 1989;161:1439–42.
5. Ueland K, Metcalfe J. Circulatory changes in pregnancy. Clin Obstet Gynecol 1975;18:41–50.
6. Laird-Meeter K, Van de Ley G, Bom TH, et al. Cardiocirculatory adjustments during pregnancy—an echocardiographic study. Clin Cardiol 1979;2:328–32.
7. Brackley KJ, Ramsay MM, Pipkin FB, et al. A longitudinal study of maternal blood-flow in normal pregnancy and the puerperium: analysis of Doppler waveforms using Laplace transform techniques. Br J Obstet Gynaecol 1998;105:68–77.
8. Bergersen TK, Hartgill TW, Pirhonen J. Cerebrovascular response to normal pregnancy: a longitudinal study. Am J Physiol Heart Circ Physiol 2006;290:H1856–61.
9. Fong J, Mack PF, Gurewitsch ED. The effect of lumbar epidural anesthesia on maternal middle cerebral artery blood flow in normal pregnancy: a prospective, randomized, double-blind comparison study. Am J Obstet Gynecol 1998;179:1237–40.
10. Rubler S, Damani PM, Pinto ER. Cardiac size and performance during pregnancy estimated with echocardiography. Am J Cardiol 1977;40:534–40.
11. Robson SC, Hunter S, Boys RJ, et al. Serial study of factors influencing changes in cardiac output during human pregnancy. Am J Physiol 1989;256:H1060–5.

12. Shotan A, Ostrzega E, Mehra A, et al. Incidence of arrhythmias in normal pregnancy and relation to palpitations, dizziness, and syncope. Am J Cardiol 1997; 79:1061–4.

13. Romem A, Romem Y, Katz M, et al. Incidence and characteristics of maternal cardiac arrhythmias during labor. Am J Cardiol 2004;93:931–3.

14. Duvekot JJ, Cheriex EC, Pieters FA, et al. Early pregnancy changes in hemodynamics and volume homeostasis are consecutive adjustments triggered by a primary fall in systemic vascular resistance. Am J Obstet Gynecol 1993;169: 1382–92.

15. Duvekot JJ, Peeters LL. Maternal cardiovascular hemodynamic adaptation to pregnancy. Obstet Gynecol Surv 1994;49:S1–14.

16. Carbillon L, Uzan M, Uzan S. Pregnancy, vascular tone, and maternal hemodynamics: a crucial adaptation. Obstet Gynecol Surv 2000;55:574–81.

17. Cutforth R, MacDonald CB. Heart sounds and murmurs in pregnancy. Am Heart J 1966;71:741–7.

18. Hendricks CH. The hemodynamics of a uterine contraction. Am J Obstet Gynecol 1958;76:969–82.

19. Adams JQ, Alexander AM. Alterations in cardiovascular physiology during labor. Obstet Gynecol 1958;12:542–9.

20. Robson SC, Dunlop W, Boys RJ, et al. Cardiac output during labour. Br Med J 1987;295:1169–72.

21. Winner W, Romney SL. Cardiovascular responses to labor and delivery. Am J Obstet Gynecol 1966;95:1104–14.

22. Ueland K, Hansen JM. Maternal cardiovascular dynamics: labor and delivery under local and caudal analgesia. Am J Obstet Gynecol 1969;103:8–18.

23. Pritchard JA. Changes in the blood volume during pregnancy and delivery. Anesthesiology 1965;26:393–9.

24. Lund CJ, Donovan JC. Blood volume during pregnancy: significance of plasma and red cell volumes. Am J Obstet Gynecol 1967;98:393–403.

25. Bernstein IM, Ziegler W, Badger GJ. Plasma volume expansion in early pregnancy. Obstet Gynecol 2001;97:669–72.

26. TJ B. Iron requirements in pregnancy and strategies to meet them. Am J Clin Nutr 2000;72(Suppl):257S–64S.

27. Heit JA, Kobbervig CE, James AH, et al. Trends in the incidence of venous thromboembolism during pregnancy or postpartum: a 30-year population-based study. Ann Intern Med 2005;143:697–706.

28. James AH, Jamison MG, Brancazio LR, et al. Venous thromboembolism during pregnancy and the postpartum period: incidence, risk factors, and mortality. Am J Obstet Gynecol 2006;194:1311–5.

29. Brenner B. Haemostatic changes in pregnancy. Thromb Res 2004;114:409–14.

30. Marik PE, Plante LA. Venous thromboembolic disease and pregnancy. N Engl J Med 2008;359:2025–33.

31. Weinberger SE, Weiss ST, Cohen WR, et al. Pregnancy and the lung. Am Rev Respir Dis 1980;121:559–81.

32. Prowse CM, Gaensler EA. Respiratory and acid-base changes during pregnancy. Anesthesiology 1965;26:381–92.

33. Elkus R, Popovich J. Respiratory physiology in pregnancy. Clin Chest Med 1992; 13:555–65.

34. McAuliffe F, Kametas N, Costello J, et al. Respiratory function in singleton and twin pregnancy. BJOG 2002;109:765–9.

35. Lucius H, Gahlenbeck H, Kleine H-O, et al. Respiratory functions, buffer system, and electrolyte concentrations of blood during human pregnancy. Respir Physiol 1970;9:311–7.
36. Thiel DH, Gavaler JS, Joshi SN, et al. Heartburn of pregnancy. Gastroenterology 1977;72:666–8.
37. Feeney JG. Heartburn in pregnancy. Br Med J 1982;284:1138–9.
38. Munnur U, de Boisblanc B, Suresh MS. Airway problems in pregnancy. Crit Care Med 2005;33(Suppl):S259–68.
39. Goldszmidt E. Principles and practice of obstetric airway management. Anesthesiol Clin 2008;26:109–25.
40. McDonnell NJ, Paech MJ, Clavisi OM, et al. Difficult and failed intubation in obstetric anesthesia: an observational study of airway management and complications associated with general anaesthesia for caesarean section. Int J Obstet Anesth 2008;17:292–7.
41. Davison JM, Dunlop W. Renal hemodynamics and tubular function in normal human pregnancy. Kidney Int 1980;18:152–61.
42. Dunlop W. Serial changes in renal hemodynamics during normal human pregnancy. BJOG 1981;88:1–9.
43. Jeyabalan A, Lain KY. Anatomic and functional changes of the upper urinary tract during pregnancy. Urol Clin North Am 2007;34:1–6.
44. Wilson M, Morganti AA, Zervoudakis I, et al. Blood pressure, the renin-aldosterone system and sex steroids throughout normal pregnancy. Am J Med 1980;68:97–104.
45. Dafnis E, Sabatini S. The effect of pregnancy on renal function: physiology and pathophysiology. Am J Med Sci 1992;303:184–205.
46. Sacks G, Sargent I, Redman C. An innate view of human pregnancy. Immunol Today 1999;114:114–8.
47. Challis JR, Lockwood CJ, Myatt L, et al. Inflammation and pregnancy. Reprod Sci 2009;16:206–15.
48. Borchers AT, Naguwa SM, Keen CL, et al. The implications of autoimmunity and pregnancy. J Autoimmun 2010;34:J287–99.
49. Nausea and vomiting of pregnancy. ACOG Practice Bulletin No. 52. American College of Obstetricians and Gynecologists. Obstet Gynecol 2004;103:803–15.
50. Frederiksen MC. Physiologic changes in pregnancy and their effect on drug disposition. Semin Perinatol 2001;25:120–3.
51. Tracy TS, Venkataramanan R, Glover DD, et al. Temporal changes in drug metabolism (CYP1A2, CYP2D6 and CYP3A activity) during pregnancy. Am J Obstet Gynecol 2005;192:633–9.
52. Pavek P, Ceckova M, Staud F. Variation of drug kinetics in pregnancy. Curr Drug Metab 2009;10:520–9.
53. Anderson GD. Pregnancy-induced changes in pharmacokinetics. Clin Pharmacokinet 2005;44:989–1008.

Imaging of Neurologic Conditions During Pregnancy and the Perinatal Period

William T. Delfyett, MD[a],*, David T. Fetzer, MD[b,c]

KEYWORDS

• Pregnancy • Radiation • Imaging • Headache • Stroke • Neuroradiology • ALARA

KEY POINTS

• The health of the mother is the most important factor in the health of the conceptus. The selection and modification of any proposed diagnostic imaging strategy should reflect this principle.
• Fetal radiation doses of less than 5 rad (50 mGy) have not been associated with an increased incidence of abnormality or pregnancy loss.
• Routine diagnostic imaging used to evaluate a pregnant patient can maintain fetal radiation doses below 5 rad (50 mGy). Radiation doses should be lowered As Low As Reasonably Achievable (ALARA) while maintaining diagnostic quality.
• Both iodinated computed tomography contrast and gadolinium-based magnetic resonance imaging contrast agents may be administered in select circumstances. However, there are few clinical questions that cannot be answered by noncontrast magnetic resonance techniques.

ANATOMY

A variety of physiologic, hormonal, immunologic, and hemodynamic changes occur throughout pregnancy.[1] Direct increases in size of the heart, kidneys, and thyroid have all been observed and generally attributed to hemodynamic and cellular changes related to hormonal influences.[2] Changes in brain size are also known to occur with the administration of high-dose exogenous steroids[3]; one specific study using

Funding sources: None.
Conflict of interest: None.
[a] Department of Radiology, UPMC Presbyterian Hospital, University of Pittsburgh School of Medicine, UPMC Presbyterian-Shadyside, 200 Lothrop Street South Tower, 8th Floor, Pittsburgh, PA 15213, USA; [b] PGY-V, UPMC Medical Graduate Program, University of Pittsburgh School of Medicine, 200 Lothrop Street, Pittsburgh, PA 15213, USA; [c] Department of Radiology, Radiology Residency Program at UPMC, 200 Lothrop Street, Suite 3950 South Tower, Pittsburgh, PA 15213, USA
* Corresponding author.
E-mail address: delfyettwt@upmc.edu

Neurol Clin 30 (2012) 791–822
http://dx.doi.org/10.1016/j.ncl.2012.06.003
0733-8619/12/$ – see front matter © 2012 Elsevier Inc. All rights reserved.

neurologic.theclinics.com

volumetric magnetic resonance imaging (MRI) demonstrated decreased brain size in both healthy and preeclamptic patients over the course of pregnancy, with return to baseline by 6 months postpartum.[4] This article briefly addresses some of the physiologic changes in pregnancy to which these anatomic changes are generally attributed, and are thus most germane to neuroimaging (**Table 1**).

During pregnancy, both the anatomy and function of the pituitary gland change significantly. Lactotroph hypertrophy leads to enlargement of the adenohypophysis during pregnancy, with up to 30% increase in gland weight and mean volume increase of 120%, as seen in **Fig. 1**.[5] The degree of enlargement is related to gestational age, with mean height of approximately 9 mm during the third trimester, up to 12 mm in the immediate postpartum period, and finally returning to a normal size by approximately 6-months postpartum.[6]

Increased levels of circulating corticotropin, prolactin, and estrogen products may have a trophic effect on neoplasms such as pituitary adenomas, hemangioblastomas, schwannomas, and meningiomas, as well as malignancies such as choriocarcinoma, melanoma, and breast carcinoma, all of which may present with intracranial metastases.[7,8] Selective immunosuppression during pregnancy, primarily from increased levels of circulating cortisol, as well as progesterone-induced T-cell inhibition, may have an inhibitory effect on autoimmune disorders such as multiple sclerosis.

The hypercoagulable state during pregnancy, caused by increased circulating fibrinogen and other clotting factors, as well as increased platelet aggregability, is compounded by the reduction in fibrinolytic activity resulting from decreased endogenous anticoagulants such as protein S and antithrombin III.[7–9] Although randomized studies have shown that there is not an increased risk of stroke during pregnancy, there is a significantly increased risk in the peripartum and immediate postpartum periods,[8,10] especially in the setting of hypertension, diabetes, hyperlipidemia, and premature atherosclerosis formation. In addition, the increased risk of arterial

Table 1
Physiologic changes in pregnancy

Hormonal	Metabolic	Immunologic	Hemodynamic	Hematologic
↑ hCG, prolactin ↑ Estrogen and progesterone precursors and products ↑ ACTH	↑ Cholesterol turnover ↑ Circulating triglycerides *(Week 20–40):* ↑ Insulin resistance; ↑ glycogen synthesis and storage	↑ Cortisol ↑ Progesterone-induced T-cell inhibitors	↑ Heart rate and stroke volume with ↑ cardiac output 40%–60% ↑ Blood volume (50% plasma and 10%–30% red cell mass resulting in pseudoanemia of pregnancy)	↑ Levels of coagulation factors (VII, IV, V, fibrinogen) ↑ Platelet aggregability ↑ Heparin neutralization ↑ Protein C inhibitors
↓ LH and FSH	*(Week 1–20):* ↓ Insulin resistance; ↓ glycogen synthesis and storage		↓ Systemic vascular resistance ↓ Blood pressure	↓ Fibrinolytic activity, antithrombin III levels ↓ Protein S inhibitor

Abbreviations: ACTH, corticotropin; FSH, follicle-stimulating hormone; hCG, human chorionic gonadotropin; LH, luteinizing hormone.

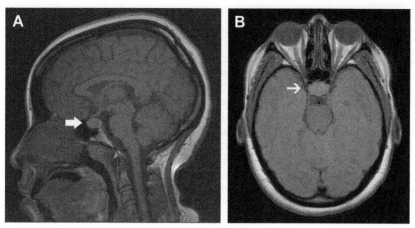

Fig. 1. A 25-year-old woman, 36 weeks pregnant, with severe headache. Physiologic hypertrophy with (*A*) Sagittal T1-weighted image demonstrating a homogeneous, enlarged pituitary gland with convex superior margin, measuring 1.2 cm in height (*large arrow*). (*B*) Axial proton-density image demonstrating a homogenously enlarged pituitary gland filling the sella (*small arrow*).

dissection or deep venous thrombosis during a prolonged or difficult labor increases the risk of embolic infarction.

Hormonal and hemodynamic changes may also be involved in the growth or development of intracranial aneurysms. Increased levels of relaxin, for example, upregulates collagenase and collagen remodeling that may affect vessel-wall integrity. The risk of subarachnoid hemorrhage (SAH), most commonly from aneurysm rupture, is 5 times greater during pregnancy than in a nonpregnant woman, and is a leading cause of maternal mortality.

IMAGING PROTOCOLS
Study Selection and Safety

The national vital statistics report for 2009 documented 4.13 million births in the United States during 2009.[11] It is estimated that there are up to 6 million pregnancies in the United States every year, with close to 2 million ending in pregnancy loss.[12] It is therefore likely that physicians across many specialties will encounter pregnant patients, including those presenting with neurologic signs or symptoms. A dilemma frequently arises in choosing the ideal imaging evaluation for the patient while attempting to reduce any potential risk for the conceptus. However, it would be regrettable if the proposed examination or evaluation algorithm were modified to such an extent that the pregnant patient was to receive poorer care than she would otherwise. Suboptimal imaging may lead to delays in treatment or even failures in diagnosis. Above all, it is clear that the health of the mother is the most important factor in the health of the fetus.

Consensus expert panels have established both practice guidelines and recommendations regarding imaging of the pregnant patient. The American College of Radiology (ACR) and the European Society of Urogenital Radiology (ESUR) have both established recommendations that have largely been in line with the official position papers from the American College of Obstetricians and Gynecologists (ACOG).[13–16] It is advisable that radiology departments develop their own official departmental policies regarding the imaging of pregnant patients, incorporating the practice guidelines of these bodies to aid physicians in the management of the pregnant patient.

Radiation Exposure

In evaluating radiation safety, one considers both deterministic and stochastic radiation effects. Deterministic effects are associated with specific threshold values of exposure, as could be achieved if multiple computed tomography (CT) examinations are performed during a single pregnancy. Deterministic effects may include organ malformations and neurologic effects such as low IQ and mental retardation. On the other hand, stochastic effects occur without any defined threshold and are believed to occur at any level of radiation. Childhood malignancies, including leukemia, are considered stochastic effects.[17,18] Given the adverse effects that can be associated with a stochastic effect, a radiation-protection paradigm has been promoted that emphasizes lowering radiation as much as possible, a principle known as ALARA (As Low As Reasonably Achievable).[13] However, radiation exposure should be balanced with image quality, and care should be taken not to lower doses to the point at which studies are no longer diagnostic.

The potential risk of ionizing radiation as it relates to adverse effects on the conceptus is known from both experimental animal studies and in utero exposures.[19–24] Long-term follow-up of the survivors of Hiroshima and Nagasaki atomic bomb explosions included 2452 survivors who were in utero at the time of the attacks and 15,388 survivors who were younger than 6 years of age. Both groups were found to have dose-related increases in solid cancers.[24] In addition, excess relative risks of leukemia have been widely reported following all types of radiation exposures.[25] Although the estimation of relative risks of leukemia vary, the dose-dependent risk has been estimated at approximately 6% per 100 rad exposure (1 Gy) in utero.[22]

Although the levels of ionizing radiation discussed here are orders of magnitude greater than would be encountered in modern diagnostic imaging, specific considerations should still be made. Exposures before 2 weeks of gestation are characterized by an "all-or-none" phenomenon in that either spontaneous loss occurs or no effect is detected. It is known that the most radiation-sensitive period for the conceptus is between 2 and 15 weeks. Commonly reported adverse effects of exposures during this time include miscarriage, growth retardation, organ malformation, and mental retardation, as well as increased risk of both solid and leukemic cancers.[13,26] Numerous studies have sought to answer the question "what radiation dose represents a safe threshold?" Unfortunately, there is as yet no clear answer.

In practice, at the most conservative level, fetal doses of less than 5 rad (50 mGy) have not been associated with an increase in fetal anomaly or pregnancy loss. The ACR practice guidelines describing the use of ionizing radiation in adolescent and potentially pregnant patients addresses potential risk in reference to this 5-rad (50 mGy) level. At fetal absorbed doses between 5 and 15 rad (150 mGy) possible potential effects may exist, but are likely too subtle to be detected clinically, especially considering 5% to 10% of births may have some form of detectable congenital defect without any history of radiation exposure.[13,27,28]

In CT the conceptus dose varies based on maternal size, examination parameters, and whether it receives direct irradiation. When interrogating a cervical spine or intracranial complaint, for example, the conceptus is far removed from direct radiation exposure; the only potential exposure would be via internal scatter radiation. Fetal dose associated with a head CT is considered to be less than 0.01 rad (0.1 mGy).[18,26,29,30] By contrast, direct irradiation could occur when performing a lumbar spine CT for maternal back pain or abdominal imaging in the setting of trauma.

Extensive research has evaluated potential fetal exposures from a variety of CT examination types and clinical indications. In these studies, a lumbar spine CT dose to the fetus is estimated at 0.28 to 2.4 rad (2.8–24 mGy) and a CT of the abdomen and pelvis may be up to 3 rad (30 mGy).[31–34]

In the clinical setting, the fetal dose cannot be measured directly; rather, an effective dose can be calculated. These calculations have been performed in several simulations for abdominopelvic CT examinations with an estimated fetal dose range from 7.3 to 14.3 mGy/100 mAs (0.73–1.4 rad/100 mAs).[35] The majority of CT scanner software can estimate the patient's radiation dose, and some vendors can provide a prospective estimate even before scanning. Advanced dose-reduction technology may be used, if available. For instance, a variety of measures exist by which the radiation exposure can be modulated, dynamically reducing doses depending on size and composition of body part.[36] In addition, varying image reconstruction techniques may offer consistent diagnostic image quality while allowing for even further reduced radiation exposure.[37–40] While these advances have made it possible to reduce radiation exposure, it is important to consider national trends of increasing CT use, including its use in the pregnant population.[41]

It is important for the radiologist to be mindful of the preset parameters of examinations as well as of dose estimates. Inclusion of the CT-scan parameters in the radiology report should be routine, and software-generated radiation dose estimates may also be included as part of the patient's medical record. These recorded data provide a means by which radiation safety officers may provide the best estimates of fetal dosages and counseling for any given patient.[42]

Magnetic Resonance

No current evidence exists that would suggest harm to the fetus exposed to magnetic fields up to 3 T. However, potential energy deposition that may cause tissue heating as well as acoustic exposure have been reported as potential concerns regarding MRI scanning. The practice guidelines of the ACR suggest deferring elective maternal examinations because of these potential concerns; however, the ACR advocates use of MRI if the results have a direct benefit to the health of the patient or fetus.[43] In fact, fetal MRI is widely used when ultrasonography cannot reliably provide diagnostic certainty. Practice guidelines for fetal MRI have been established jointly by the ACR and the Society of Pediatric Radiology (SPR).[44]

Contrast Administration

The intravenous administration of iodinated CT contrast agents to the pregnant patient has not been associated with any teratogenic effect; however, some studies have raised concerns for neonatal hypothyroidism. Therefore, intravenous contrast administration should be deferred during pregnancy when possible. For examinations such as CT venography or arteriography for which contrast is required, written informed consent should be obtained, and subsequent attention is warranted during neonatal screening for hypothyroidism, already a component of many state and governmentally mandated newborn screening programs.[14,45]

The administration of gadolinium-based MRI contrast agents should be deferred during pregnancy whenever possible. Gadolinium chelates have been shown to cross the placental barrier, enter fetal circulation, and pass into the amniotic fluid by renal excretion before being completely eliminated. Animal studies have demonstrated developmental abnormalities following gadolinium exposure, albeit at concentrations far higher than would be used in clinical settings. Given the lack of evidence regarding the clinical range of dosages, administration may be performed when clinically warranted. If noncontrast MR techniques are not considered adequate in specific clinical scenarios, signed informed consent should be obtained following a well-documented risk-benefit analysis.[43]

Some iodinated contrast agents are passed into breast milk. Similarly, extremely small amounts of gadolinium-based agents are excreted into breast milk, but these have not been associated with any adverse outcomes. The ACOG and ACR guidelines do not advocate any interruption of breastfeeding following administration of iodinated contrast nor following gadolinium contrast administration.[16] The European Society of Urogenital Radiology differs from the ACOG and ACR on this point, advocating a 24-hour interruption of breastfeeding following the administration of a gadolinium agent.[15] A period of interruption of breastfeeding ("pump and dump") may be offered as an option to allay maternal concern.

PATHOLOGY
Vascular

Subarachnoid hemorrhage
SAH during pregnancy is 5 times more likely than in the nonpregnant population, with a prevalence of 1 in every 10,000 patients (0.01%–0.05%), and is the third leading cause of nonobstetric-related maternal death.[10] Primigravida, increased maternal age, and advanced gestation age convey even greater risk.[46] The increased risk may relate to the increased circulating relaxin and the upregulation of collagen remodeling.[7] As in the nonpregnant population, patients present with acute onset of severe headache and meningismus. The most common cause of SAH, also as in the nonpregnant patient, is rupture of an intracranial aneurysm, typically emanating from the circle of Willis.[8,47]

Noncontrast CT is the first-line examination with sensitivity greater than 90%, and remains the preferred modality to follow up intraparenchymal extension and hydrocephalus.[10] Catheter angiography remains the gold standard; however, CT angiography also offers rapid and noninvasive interrogation of the intracranial vasculature, and may be used for treatment planning. However, when readily available, MRI should be considered. MR angiography offers noncontrast techniques, using 3-dimensional time-of-flight imaging, allowing for the assessment and follow-up of nonruptured aneurysms without radiation exposure. Important findings include aneurysm size, location, and additional characteristics such as neck size (narrow vs wide mouth), proximity to vessel origins, and orientation of the aneurysm apex in relation to its base.

Studies have shown that treatment of ruptured aneurysms is beneficial to both mother and fetus (52% reduction and 22% reduction in mortality rates, respectively). Both endovascular coiling and surgical clipping may be attempted, depending on aneurysm size, location, and other characteristics. For incidentally identified unruptured aneurysms, treatment is typically considered for symptomatic or enlarging lesions.[47] Debate exists regarding delivery options, with cesarean section typically recommended to decrease the risk of increasing intracranial pressure during labor and delivery; however, incidence of rupture of untreated or incompletely treated aneurysms between vaginal and cesarean delivery are not significantly different and are similar to that of the background population.

Primary nonaneurysmal SAH is a diagnosis of exclusion. Rarely SAH may be identified by noncontrast CT or lumbar puncture with no aneurysm identified, even by catheter angiography. Nonaneurysmal SAH is typically induced by hypertension, and may relate to failure of intracranial autoregulation and rupture of the relatively thin-walled pial veins.[48] Spinal MRI may be attempted, and repeat cerebral catheter angiography may be considered.

Stroke and venous thrombosis

Despite the physiologic changes associated with pregnancy, multicenter randomized trials have not shown an increased risk of ischemic or hemorrhagic infarction during pregnancy. In the first several weeks following delivery, however, the risk of infarction is markedly increased. The imaging findings of acute stroke and ischemic syndromes are essentially unchanged whether the patient is pregnant or not (**Table 2**).

Although pregnancy is a hypercoagulable state, the risk of cerebral venous thrombosis (CVT) is greatest in the first 2 to 4 weeks following delivery (**Fig. 2**). CVT is reported to account for up to 6% of maternal deaths, so prompt diagnosis and initiation of therapy is essential. Common presenting symptoms include headache, seizure, papilledema, encephalopathy, focal neurologic deficit, and symptoms mimicking idiopathic intracranial hypertension (IIH). In the evaluation of any patient with suspected elevated intracranial pressure, CVT is an important factor to consider, as intracranial hypertension may be observed in up to 20% to 40% of patients with CVT. Venous thrombosis is also an important potential cause of parenchymal hemorrhage (**Fig. 3**). Venous infarctions tend to be peripheral, do not respect arterial territories, and may involve deep brain structures bilaterally (**Fig. 4**). Outflow obstruction occurs with venous thrombosis and if collateral drainage is inadequate, the increase in venous pressure may overcome arterial perfusion pressure, causing an infarction. Variability in the degree of collateral drainage as well as the consideration that thromboses may partially recanalize contribute to the occasional waxing and waning of symptoms, parenchymal changes, and the simultaneous occurrence of both vasogenic and cytotoxic edema.[49–52]

CT and MRI techniques are the most widely used in the evaluation of suspected CVT. Digital-subtraction catheter angiography remains the gold standard and will likely be used in especially troublesome cases.

The most common direct sign of venous sinus thrombosis on noncontrast CT is a focal hyperdense venous sinus, but this is actually only seen in a minority of cases, reportedly up to 25%.[53] Dehydration, elevated hematocrit, adjacent hemorrhage, motion, or streak artifact are potential pitfalls, and could cause the spurious appearance of a hyperdense venous structure. Other potential noncontrast CT findings associated with venous thrombosis may include cerebral edema, focal areas of cytotoxic or vasogenic edema, parenchymal hemorrhage, subdural hemorrhage, or findings suggestive of IIH; however, noncontrast CT may be normal.[54] Any suspected hyperdense venous structure would warrant further evaluation.

Considerable anatomic variation exists in the pattern of superficial draining veins as well as of the dural venous sinuses.[55] These normal anatomic factors could contribute to potential pitfalls and errors in diagnosis, regardless of whether using CT venography or MR venographic techniques, and are listed in **Box 1**.

CT venography is an increasingly available tool to quickly evaluate patients with suspected venous thrombosis. Focal venous cutoffs or filling defects in an otherwise enhancing dural sinus are common findings of venous thrombosis. A classic finding is the "empty-delta" sign, thrombus as a low-attenuation filling defect within the superior sagittal sinus seen in cross section (see **Fig. 2A, B**). Streak artifact and beam hardening from the adjacent inner table of the skull may reduce sensitivity of CT venography when interrogating small cortical veins, for which MR blood-sensitive techniques are generally superior (see **Figs. 3C and 4C**).[66]

MRI is often the preferred method of evaluating suspected CVT in pregnancy. Both anatomic and venographic MR evaluations are used to maximize sensitivity and specificity (see **Figs. 2–4**). The brain parenchymal changes associated with CVT will be more readily apparent on MRI, and the venous sinuses can be evaluated by both anatomic and venographic techniques.

Table 2
Imaging findings in acute stroke

	Hyperacute Stroke	Acute Stroke	Early Subacute Stroke	Late Subacute Stroke	Chronic Stroke
Noncontrast CT	Possibly normal Identification and exclusion of intracranial hemorrhage Hypoattenuating Gray matter (loss of gray-white differentiation) Mass effect Hyperattenuating artery indicating vascular thrombosis	Progressive hypoattenuation of involved parenchyma, vasogenic edema visible by 12 h Progressive mass effect Exclusion of hemorrhagic transformation	Progressive mass effect, vasogenic edema and mass effect peak at 3–5 d	Resolution of mass effect	Encephalomalacia
Diffusion MRI	Possibly normal Restricted diffusion as early as 1 h	Restricted diffusion of affected parenchyma	DWI remains elevated signal, ADC normalizes over 5–7 d	DWI elevated signal resolves over approximately 4 wk	Encephalomalacia Possible cortical laminar necrosis
T2-weighted and FLAIR MRI	Normal or minimal signal change Possibly loss in flow voids indicating vascular thrombus or slow flow Possible elevated vascular FLAIR signal indicating thrombosis or sluggish flow	Elevated FLAIR signal after 4 h Early mass effect	Elevated FLAIR and T2 Mass effect peaks along with CT	Mass effect resolves	Encephalomalacia

Abbreviations: ADC, apparent diffusion coefficient; CT, computed tomography; DWI, diffusion-weighted imaging; FLAIR, fluid-attenuated inversion recovery; MRI, magnetic resonance imaging.

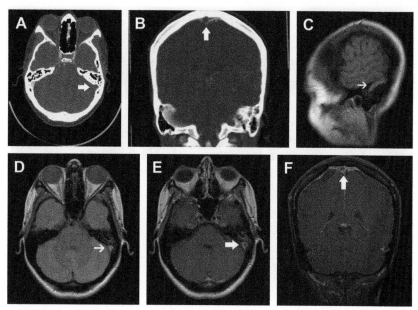

Fig. 2. A 27-year-old woman, 3 weeks postpartum, with history of preeclampsia, presenting with headaches. Superior sagittal and transverse venous sinus thrombosis seen on (*A*) axial and (*B*) sagittal CT venogram with dural venous filling defect (*large arrow*). (*C*) Coronal T1-weighted MRI and (*D*) axial proton-density imaging demonstrate loss of normal flow void and intrinsic T1 hyperintensity (*small arrow*). (*E*) Axial and (*F*) sagittal postcontrast MRI also demonstrate venous sinus filling defects (*large arrow*).

Each specific MRI venographic technique has its potential pitfalls and limitations, which are all important to consider. On routine MRI anatomic imaging using T1- and T2-weighted sequences, for example, the venous sinuses appear as flow voids, the loss of which could be consistent with thrombosis or slow flow (see **Figs. 2**C and **3**A). Slow or turbulent flow is a potential mimic of thrombosis, and can occur normally or in the setting of a recanalized, partially thrombosed sinus.[52] Furthermore, the signal intensity of venous thrombus varies with age, likely attributable to paramagnetic effects of the varying hemoglobin breakdown products.[52,67–69]

Gradient-recall echo (GRE) and T2*-weighted sequences are particularly sensitive to blood products. The abnormal blooming artifact produced on GRE sequences from paramagnetic blood products is especially helpful in acute cases of thrombosis, particularly when T1 and T2 signal abnormalities may be inconclusive (see **Fig. 4**C). These sequences, as well as specific blood-sensitive, susceptibility-weighted sequences, have also been shown to be helpful in the identification of thromboses of small cortical veins (see **Fig. 3**C).[66,68]

Dural venous thrombosis can have a varied appearance on diffusion-weighted imaging (DWI), including both elevated and decreased signal. Elevated DWI signal in a thrombosed sinus with associated decreased apparent diffusion coefficient (ADC) may be seen in only up to 41% of cases.[67,70,71] Parenchymal changes with CVT may also be varied on DWI, reflecting the possible combination of facilitated diffusion (vasogenic edema) and restricted diffusion (cytotoxic edema).[50]

Careful evaluation of a variety of sequences can overcome many of these difficulties, but supplementing the evaluation with MR venography is suggested. A variety

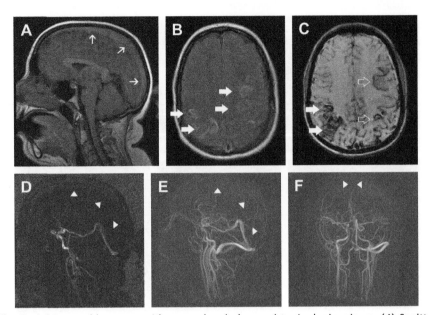

Fig. 3. A 24-year-old woman with severe headaches and tonic-clonic seizure. (*A*) Sagittal T1-weighted image with loss of flow void and intrinsic T1 hyperintensity involving the superior sagittal sinus (*small arrows*). Physiologic pituitary hypertrophy is also demonstrated. (*B*) Axial fluid-attenuated inversion recovery (FLAIR) image demonstrates bilateral frontoparietal cortical and subcortical areas of signal abnormality (*large arrows*). (*C*) Susceptibility-weighted imaging shows corresponding areas of blooming artifact, representing areas of hemorrhage (*large arrows*), while serpiginous areas of signal loss likely represent thrombosed or slow flow within cortical veins (*open arrows*). (*D*) Two-dimensional phase-contrast imaging demonstrates lack of flow-related signal within the superior sagittal sinus (*arrowheads*). (*E*, *F*) Three-dimensional time-of-flight imaging with similar findings (*arrowheads*).

of techniques may be employed to obtain MR venographic images, all of which maximize the signal obtained from the dural venous sinuses and minimize the parenchymal signal, ideally to identify areas of filling defects. Most commonly either phase-contrast (see **Fig. 3**D) or time-of-flight (see **Fig. 3**E, F) techniques are used to evaluate the pregnant patient, as they can both be performed without contrast. With MR venography,

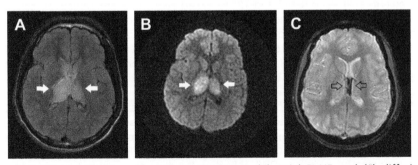

Fig. 4. A 22-year-old man with new-onset seizures. (*A*) Axial FLAIR and (*B*) diffusion-weighted imaging (DWI) demonstrate venous infarction of the bilateral thalami (*large arrows*). (*C*) Axial gradient-recall echo demonstrates blooming artifact within the internal cerebral veins, representing thrombosis (*open arrows*).

Box 1
Anatomic features or variants that may cause potential pitfalls in CT venography and MR venography
Left/right asymmetry of transverse sinuses (up to 40% of cases)
Variant branching at the torcula simulating a filling defect
Variant patterns of tributary veins
Venous septations
Arachnoid granulations appearing as small filling defects
Arachnoid granulations exceeding 1 cm in size, not following cerebrospinal fluid signal
Data from Refs.[56-65]

however, gaps in the apparent flow may be noted in up to 31% of normal cases, which may be due to venous septations, turbulent flow, or the angle of slice selection.[72] Specific aspects of these techniques that potentially affect diagnoses of thrombosis are summarized in **Table 3**.

The administration of contrast may increase diagnostic sensitivity and specificity of MR venography, and a variety of techniques have been described.[73-75] Given the potential concern regarding contrast administration in the pregnant patient, these should be reserved for the postpartum period.

Parenchymal Abnormalities

Preeclampsia

Preeclampsia is a complex clinical condition/syndrome affecting 5% to 10% of all pregnancies (up to 30% of twin gestations) and is defined by the presence of

Table 3
Potential pitfalls of venographic techniques

Type of Potential Pitfalls	CT Venogram	Phase-Contrast MRV	Time-of-Flight MRV	Contrast-Enhanced MRV
Technical	Streak artifact and beam hardening along inner table Poor opacification of venous system related to contrast administration	Longer imaging times, potential for patient motion User-defined velocity encoding and possibility of aliasing artifact Lower spatial resolution than TOF Smaller anatomic coverage than TOF	Maximal signal obtained perpendicular to plane of acquisition in plane saturation slow and turbulent flow T1 signal from thrombus mimicking flow	Need for gadolinium-based contrast agents

Abbreviations: MRV, magnetic resonance venography; TOF, time-of-flight.
   Data from Ayanzen RH, Bird CR, Keller PJ, et al. Cerebral MR venography: normal anatomy, and potential diagnostic pitfalls. AJNR Am J Neuroradiol 2000;21:74–8; and Provenzale JM, Joseph GJ, Barborial DP. Dural sinus thrombosis: findings on CT and MR imaging and diagnostic pitfalls. AJR Am J Roentgenol 1998;170:777–83.

hypertension, proteinuria, and peripheral edema, typically presenting around the 20th week of gestation.[10,76] Specific etiology is unknown; however, some theorize that a placental-derived toxin contributes to widespread vascular derangements, disruption of autoregulation, and breakdown of the blood-brain barrier. Patients may present clinically with headaches, visual disturbances, confusion, and right upper quadrant pain. There is also increased risk of intracranial hemorrhage and vasospasm; however, findings typically resolve shortly following delivery of the placenta.

If the patient presents with seizures or coma, the diagnosis of eclampsia is made. This life-threatening condition is treated medically with hypertension control and seizure prophylaxis with magnesium sulfate; however, if seizure activity persists, emergent delivery may be required. Patients may also present with hemolytic anemia, elevated liver function tests, and low platelet count, part of the HELLP syndrome; thrombocytopenia may predispose patients to cerebral hemorrhage.[77]

In patients with preeclampsia/eclampsia, patients may present clinically with hypertensive encephalopathy, identical to findings seen with posterior reversible encephalopathy syndrome (PRES), also known as reversible posterior leukoencephalopathy syndrome (RPLS).[8,77] Although the etiology remains unknown, PRES/RPLS is believed to be multifactorial and involve circulating cytotoxic factors, leading to disruptions in cerebral autoregulation, increased vascular endothelium permeability, and vasogenic edema.[77] PRES is also associated with systemic lupus erythematosus (SLE) and thrombotic thrombocytopenic purpura (TTP), and is seen in patients receiving cyclosporine, tacrolimus, and chemotherapy. In pregnancy, it typically occurs during the third trimester and during the 6- to 8-week postpartum period. Patients may present with self-limited severe headache, seizures, and cortical blindness, which may also be accompanied by vasospasm and intracranial hemorrhage.[7]

Imaging findings of eclampsia and hypertensive encephalopathy may also be identical to PRES/RPLS.[8] CT findings are nonspecific with areas of patchy white matter hypoattenuation. Watershed regions are the most affected, particularly in the occipital regions; however, the frontal and parietal lobes may also be involved (**Fig. 5**).[10] On CT,

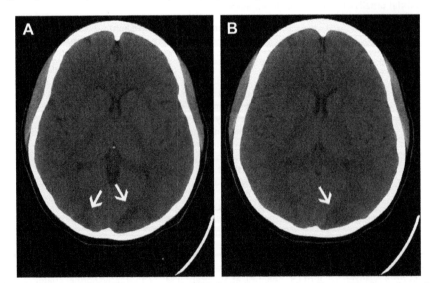

Fig. 5. A 28-year-old pregnant woman with hypertension presenting with altered mental status, diagnosed with eclampsia. (*A, B*) Noncontrast CT images demonstrate patchy areas of cortical and subcortical white matter hypoattenuation (*arrows*).

areas of hyperattenuation likely signify subarachnoid or even parenchymal hemorrhage. On MRI, patchy areas of T1 hypointensity and T2 hyperintensity affect the subcortical parieto-occipital regions, and may also involve the frontal lobes, basal ganglia, pons, and brainstem; cortical involvement may also be seen (**Figs. 6** and **7**); the T2 signal abnormalities may be most conspicuous on fluid-attenuated inversion recovery (FLAIR) sequences. Hemorrhage may occur (**Fig. 8**), and variable enhancement is also a known imaging finding.[10] Facilitated diffusion may result in increased signal on DWI and would correspond to areas of increased pixel values on ADC maps; true areas of parenchymal infarction may occur and would demonstrate decreased values on ADC maps. Angiography may demonstrate vasospasm of the medium and large cerebral arteries, particularly involving the basilar artery (see **Fig. 6**E, F).

Postpartum angiopathy

Postpartum angiopathy (PCA), also known as peripartum cerebral angiopathy or vasculopathy, is indistinguishable from eclampsia and PRES/RPLS on imaging. Clinically PCA also presents with severe headaches, seizures, and focal neurologic deficits, but occurs in normotensive women without proteinuria, typically in the 4-week postpartum period.[7,78,79] Clinical information is often required to differentiate these diagnoses; however, some investigators believe that PCA, eclampsia, hypertensive encephalopathy, and PRES/RPLS are different manifestations of the same underlying pathophysiologic process. The idiopathic form of PCA is typically reversible and nonrelapsing.[8] An iatrogenic form of PCA has been linked to the administration of bromocriptine (lactation suppression), ergot alkaloids (postpartum hemorrhage), and sympathomimetics (often found in cold medication and nasal decongestants).[8,80] Imaging features are similar to those of PRES, with patchy T2 hyperintense white matter lesions in the watershed areas (see **Fig. 8**; **Fig. 9**). Catheter angiography may demonstrate

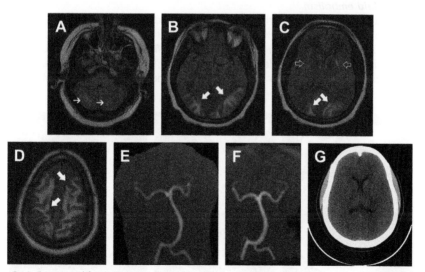

Fig. 6. A 21-year-old postpartum woman with hypertensive episode and new right-sided weakness. (*A–D*) Axial FLAIR images demonstrate cerebellar (*small arrows*), subcortical white matter (*large arrows*), and basal ganglia (*open arrows*) signal abnormalities. Three-dimensional time-of-flight angiography with maximum intensity before (*E*) and after (*F*) the neurologic symptoms shows mild narrowing and irregularity of the basilar artery during the hypertensive crisis. (*G*) A follow up head CT 3 months later was normal.

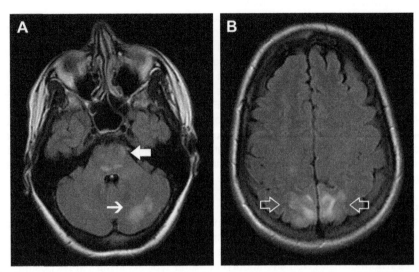

Fig. 7. A 38-year-old woman, 6 days following cesarean section, with hypertensive episode and seizures. (*A, B*) Axial FLAIR images demonstrate cerebellar (*small arrow*), pons (*large arrow*), and cortical/subcortical (*open arrows*) signal abnormalities.

multifocal and reversible stenoses (arterial beading), primarily within the anterior circulation. Treatment is typically supportive, steroids are often provided, and intracranial angioplasty is rarely required. Infarction and intracranial hemorrhage may also be seen rarely.

Amniotic fluid embolism

Amniotic fluid embolism is a fairly rare entity with incidence of about 1 in 20,000 deliveries, accounting for 5% to 10% of maternal mortality in the United States. Mortality reaches 60%, and most survivors suffer from significant neurologic morbidity. The pathophysiology is poorly understood; however, it is believed to require ruptured membranes, breach of uterine or cervical veins, and a pressure gradient between

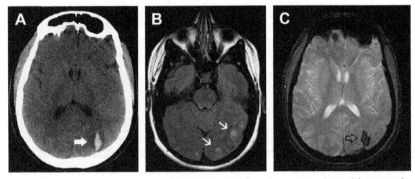

Fig. 8. A 28-year-old woman, 33 weeks pregnant with twins, presenting with severe headache. (*A*) Noncontrast CT demonstrates an area of hemorrhage within the left occipital lobe (*large arrow*). (*B*) FLAIR image shows areas of cortical/subcortical signal abnormalities (*small arrows*). (*C*) Gradient-echo imaging demonstrates blood product–related bloom artifact (*open arrow*).

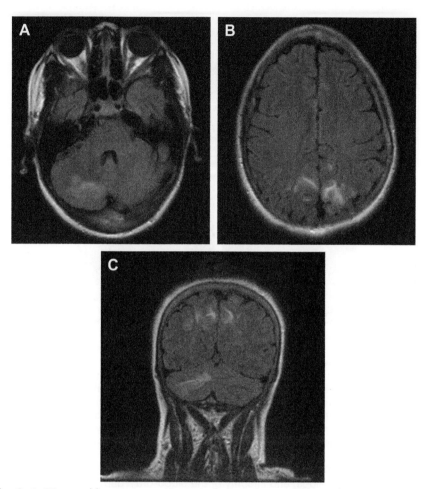

Fig. 9. A 35-year-old woman, postpartum from twin gestation and cesarean section, without history of prepartum or gestational hypertension, presenting with tonic-clonic seizure. (*A, B*) Axial and (*C*) coronal FLAIR images demonstrate subcortical white matter signal alterations. Presumptive diagnosis was postpartum angiopathy, given the normotensive state.

the uterus and venous drainage, allowing for passage of amniotic fluid, fetal cells, and other debris into the maternal circulation. Cardiorespiratory collapse may ensue, with the patient clinically presenting with anaphylaxis, leading some to suggest the term anaphylactoid syndrome of pregnancy. Imaging findings are nonspecific with areas of restricted diffusion and associated vasogenic edema within multiple vascular territories, suggesting an embolic event (**Fig. 10**).

Wernicke encephalopathy

Wernicke encephalopathy is a potentially life-threatening condition resulting from severe deficiency in thiamine.[81] Most frequently, Wernicke encephalopathy occurs in the setting of alcoholism and associated malnutrition, although it can occur in other conditions including hyperemesis gravidarum in pregnancy. In the setting of severe

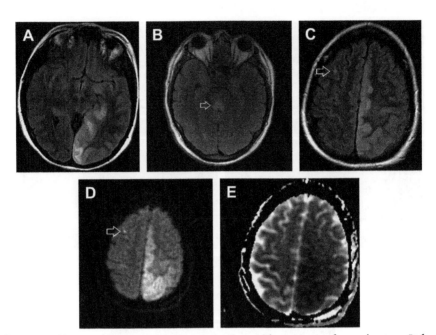

Fig. 10. A 33-year-old woman, term, presenting with rupture of membranes. Before delivery, the patient went into cardiovascular collapse and cardiac arrest. Emergency cesarean section was performed. The patient suffered from pulmonary edema, disseminated intravascular coagulation, and multiorgan failure; (*A–C*) FLAIR images show areas of cortical and white matter signal abnormality within the right occipital, parietal, parafalcine frontal, and mesial temporal regions. (*D*) Associated diffusion abnormality with (*E*) corresponding signal drop of apparent diffusion coefficient maps represents areas of acute infarction. A single focus of infarction is also identified on the contralateral side (*open arrow*). Amniotic embolism was suspected clinically, explaining the constellation of acute findings.

deficiency, neuron metabolism is impaired, lactic acid accumulation ensues, an osmotic gradient develops, and integrity of the blood-brain barrier may be impaired. This abnormality is prone to occur in regions where thiamine-dependent glucose metabolism is highest, accounting for the fairly distinct appearance on MRI. Wernicke encephalopathy is characterized by an abnormally elevated T2 signal at the medial thalami, mammillary bodies, periaqueductal gray matter, floor of the fourth ventricle, and superior cerebellar vermis (**Fig. 11**). Restricted diffusion on DWI may also be seen, along with abnormal enhancement of the affected structures following contrast administration.

Although most cases described are in the setting of alcoholism and malnourishment, consideration of this diagnosis and the recognition of the fairly characteristic imaging findings may facilitate a prompt diagnosis and early initiation of life-saving therapy in patient populations where the diagnosis might not otherwise be suspected clinically.

Multiple sclerosis

The relative ratio of female to male incidence of multiple sclerosis (MS) varies by region, ranging from 2:1 to 3:1, and has possibly been increasing over the past 60 years.[82] Given the incidence of MS in reproductive-age women, it should not be unexpected that women with MS may present for neurologic imaging while pregnant or in the postpartum period. The underlying pathogenesis of MS has not been fully

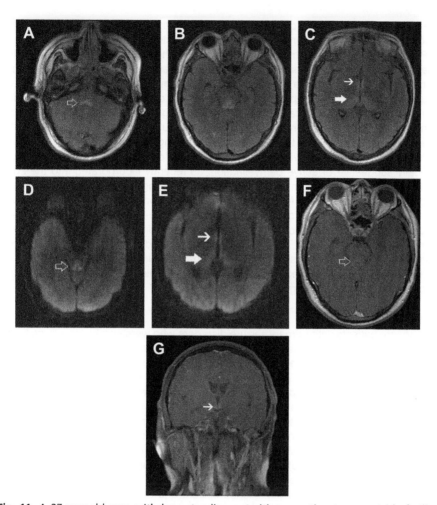

Fig. 11. A 27-year-old man with long-standing enteritis presenting to an outside facility with dizziness and abdominal pain. A rapid decline in neurologic status necessitated transfer. On arrival he was found to be unresponsive, with diffuse slowing on electroencephalogram. FLAIR images demonstrate abnormal signal in (*A*) floor of the fourth ventricle and (*B*) periaqueductal gray (*open arrow*), (*C*) medial thalami (*large arrow*) and mammillary bodies (*small arrow*). (*D, E*) DWI shows associated restricted diffusion at periaqueductal gray matter (*open arrow*), medial thalami (*large arrow*), mamillary bodies/hypothalamus (*small arrow*). (*F, G*) Postcontrast T1-weighted image demonstrates associated enhancement at periaqueductal gray matter (*open arrow*), anteromedial thalami (*arrow*). Subsequent autopsy revealed macrophage-rich infiltrate involving the periaqueductal brainstem, medial thalamus, hypothalamus, and mammillary bodies, consistent with acute Wernicke encephalopathy.

elucidated. As already discussed, in pregnancy estrogen and progesterone increase until delivery, and normalize during the postpartum period. Considering the immunologic cascade pertinent to MS, as well as varied effects of pregnancy hormones, it has been proposed that pregnancy may offer an immunosuppressive effect.[83–85] Studies have reported that the relapse rate of MS decreases during pregnancy, especially during the third trimester, and that a return to normal or even rebound relapses may occur postpartum.[86] A large area of study in MS and pregnancy has been evaluating the safety and efficacy of disease-modulating treatments during pregnancy, a full discussion of which is beyond the scope of this article.

Performance of a noncontrast brain or spinal MRI should be considered the first-line imaging choice for the pregnant MS patient who presents with new or changing symptoms, with little if any role for CT. Abnormal plaques on FLAIR or T2-weighted sequences may be readily apparent, and new lesions can be identified on comparison with prior examinations. In cases of possible new diagnoses of MS or other demyelinating syndromes during pregnancy, lesion distribution and number can still be assessed with noncontrast techniques when applying diagnostic criteria.[87,88] These noncontrast examinations would not allow for detection of the enhancing MS plaque, typically suggestive of active demyelination, as recently incorporated into the 2010 revision of the McDonald criteria.[88–90] However, as suggested in the ACR guidance document regarding safe MR practices, the decision to administer exogenous gadolinium-based contrast should be made on a case-by-case basis, after a well-documented consideration of both risks and benefits, including the referring physician, interpreting radiologist, and the patient, who should complete relevant informed consent documentation. Aside from decisions surrounding the administration of contrast, the MRI of the pregnant patient with MS would not vary from the imaging approaches used in nonpregnant patients.

Epilepsy/seizure

In pregnant patients with primary seizure disorders who were enrolled in a large European registry (EURAP), baseline seizure control was maintained without change in symptoms in 63.6% of women, with approximately 93% being seizure free throughout pregnancy. Approximately 17% and 16% of women had increases and decreases in their seizure frequency, respectively.[91] Although most women with epilepsy experience no change in seizure activity, there are conflicting reports regarding incidence and treatment during pregnancy.[92–94] There are known potential teratogenic effects of a variety of antiepileptic drugs (AEDs), with various drug classes and dosages influencing teratogenic potential.[95–97] Balancing the risks of various classes of AED therapy with those associated with uncontrolled seizures should be the primary management dilemma, rather than imaging.

There is little need to alter established seizure and epilepsy MRI protocols when considering a pregnant patient. Thin-section volumetric acquisition of T1-weighted sequences allows for detailed evaluation of anatomy, cortical gyral patterns, and detection of heterotopic gray matter. T2-weighted and FLAIR sequences may be used without modification for evaluation of hippocampal, mesial temporal, and other parenchymal signal abnormalities. In established patients, MRI evaluation is most frequently performed without contrast.

In cases where administration of gadolinium-based contrast is desired, the decision returns to a careful consideration of risk versus benefit. For example, in a pregnant patient newly presenting with seizure, administration of gadolinium contrast may be desirable as part of an initial workup. While a primary seizure disorder could present during pregnancy, a host of other potential causes of seizure would have to be considered, including, though not limited to, the possibility of meningitis, encephalitis, inflammatory parenchymal changes, metastatic disease, and underlying parenchymal lesions, for all of which contrast administration would be beneficial but not essential. Potential venous thrombosis can also be evaluated with contrast-enhanced CT or a host of noncontrast MR techniques.[52] Only in a minority of cases will a definitive diagnosis for an underlying cause of seizure prove troublesome, at which time the decision of whether to administer gadolinium-based contrast will be considered.

Neoplasm: gestational trophoblastic disease

There are several types of pregnancy-related malignancies that range from the benign hydatidiform molar to invasive molar pregnancy, with the most aggressive subset being choriocarcinoma, an aggressive and highly invasive vascular tumor. These conditions are rare and rates of incidence vary worldwide, with choriocarcinoma incidence ranging from 2 to 202 per 100,000 pregnancies.[98] In addition to local disease, choriocarcinoma may metastasize to the brain, spine, liver, and lungs. Choriocarcinoma metastases to the brain frequently present as a hemorrhagic lesion or as a frank intracranial hemorrhage.[99,100] The appearance of choriocarcinoma brain metastases on CT frequently includes parenchymal hyperdense lesions with associated edema. The MR appearance may include elevated T1 signal indicating the presence of methemoglobin, variable T2 signal, and abnormal susceptibility artifact on GRE or T2*-weighted sequences. Similar to the evaluation for other hemorrhagic metastases, inclusion of these blood product–sensitive sequences may reveal tiny foci of disease that are relatively occult on other sequences because of their small size.

Neoplasm: trophic effect of pregnancy

The hormonal changes of pregnancy are known to have a potential trophic effect on a variety of neoplasms throughout the central nervous system, including meningiomas, ependymomas (**Fig. 12**), hemangioblastomas, pituitary adenomas, and schwannomas. Similar trophic effects have also been reported for metastatic disease such as melanoma or breast carcinoma.

Pituitary and Parasellar Abnormalities

It is a normal physiologic finding for the pituitary to develop a convex superior margin during pregnancy, as opposed to the usual concave upper margin in the normal, nonpregnant adult. This expected physiologic change could mimic the radiologic appearance of pituitary hyperplasia in the nonpregnant patient, and though this is usually asymptomatic, mass effect may cause optic chiasmal compression and present clinically with bitemporal hemianopsia.

Sheehan syndrome/pituitary apoplexy

Sheehan syndrome describes the acute onset or occasionally indolent clinical manifestation of pituitary hypothalamic dysfunction related to pituitary ischemia and necrosis.[5] This ischemic event may occur secondary to maternal hypotension, frequently related to obstetric hemorrhage at or around the time of delivery; however, any cause of hypotension or shock may be a precipitating factor. Acutely, MR evaluation may demonstrate an enlarged pituitary gland without evidence of hemorrhage. Over time, involution of the gland occurs and the sella may have a partially or completely "empty" appearance on both CT and MRI (**Fig. 13**).

Pituitary apoplexy is an acute hemorrhagic infarction of the pituitary that may present similarly to a nonhemorrhagic infarction and Sheehan syndrome[5,101] However, acutely the rapid pituitary enlargement is accompanied by hemorrhage and may be associated with sudden onset of severe headache, nausea, vomiting, visual changes relating to upward mass effect on the optic chiasm, and other cranial neuropathies. An initial evaluation with head CT may potentially demonstrate hemorrhage within an enlarged pituitary, although pituitary enlargement may be seen without definite hemorrhage; it is important to consider obtaining an MRI in these cases as pituitary hemorrhage and enlargement may be missed on a routine CT scan. The MRI appearance of blood products will vary on both T1- and T2-weighted imaging according to the stage of blood-product breakdown, an aspect that is always important to consider when evaluating cases of suspected hemorrhage (**Fig. 14**).

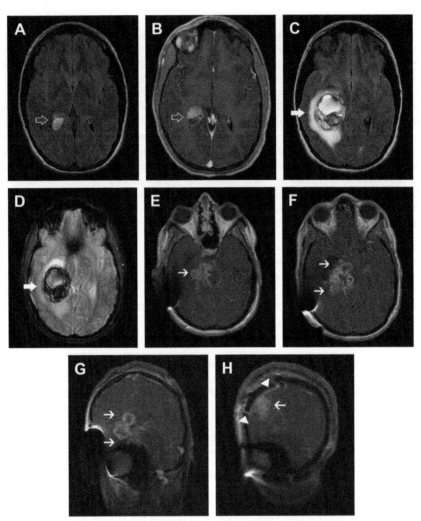

Fig. 12. An 18-year-old woman presenting with loss of consciousness. (*A*) Axial FLAIR and (*B*) postcontrast T1-weighted images demonstrate a lobulated, enhancing periventricular mass adjacent to the right atrium (*open arrow*). Diagnosis of ependymoma was made by subsequent biopsy. Five months later, approximately 10 weeks pregnant, the patient presented with neck pain and seizure activity. (*C*) Axial FLAIR and (*D*) gradient-echo images demonstrate interval enlargement of and hemorrhage into the right periventricular mass (*large arrow*). Twenty weeks later, at 30 weeks' gestation, an emergency cesarean section was performed owing to seizures and uncontrolled hypertension. Subsequent contrast-enhanced MRI (*E–H*) demonstrates dramatic interval enlargement with superior and infratentorial extension (including to midbrain) (*small arrows*) and carcinomatosis (*arrowheads*).

Pituitary tumors

Tumors of the pituitary gland can be classified by size as either microadenoma (<10 mm) or macroadenoma (>10 mm). Medical therapy is an option for these slow-growing tumors, although surgical resection or debulking may be required in patients presenting with visual-field abnormalities or symptoms relating to direct invasion of

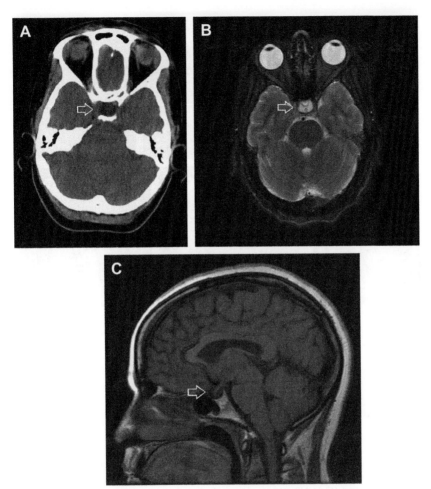

Fig. 13. A 37-year-old woman, 15 years postpartum, with chronic glucocorticoid and thyroid hormone deficiency; (*A*) Noncontrast CT, (*B*) axial FLAIR, and (*C*) sagittal T1-weighted images demonstrate a cerebrospinal fluid–filled, empty sella (*open arrow*). The infundibulum is normally positioned, suggesting the absence of a space-occupying cystic lesion.

adjacent structures. Chiasmal compression, local invasion, and significant enlargement were found during pregnancy in up to 20% of pregnant patients with macroadenomas in one series (**Fig. 15**). Microadenomas more frequently have a benign course, with only up to 5% of pregnant patients reporting increases in headaches during pregnancy and only 1% presenting with visual-field changes.[101]

Microadenomas and macroadenomas appear as discrete mass lesions intrinsic to the pituitary gland. These lesions often demonstrate gadolinium contrast enhancement, which is less avid than the remainder or the pituitary gland, appearing as a low-signal area within the gland. A subset of tumors may enhance rather rapidly and appear less conspicuously on postcontrast thin-section imaging. In these cases a dynamic contrast-enhanced series with both early and delayed enhancement acquisitions may be obtained to aid in lesion detection.

Other parasellar lesions also deserve attention. The possibility for accelerated growth of meningiomas during pregnancy is well known. Anatomically, meningiomas

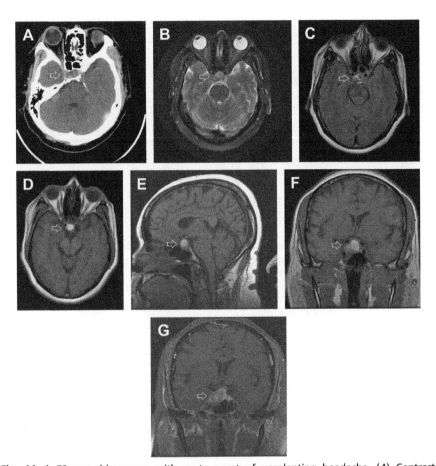

Fig. 14. A 59-year-old woman with acute onset of unrelenting headache. (*A*) Contrast-enhanced CT demonstrates an expanded sella with areas of nodular enhancement (*open arrow*). (*B*) T2-weighted and (*C*) FLAIR images demonstrate a heterogenous intrasellar signal (*open arrows*) while (*D*) axial and (*E*) sagittal, and (*F*) coronal precontrast T1-weighted images demonstrate intrinsic T1 hyperintensity suggesting hemorrhage (*open arrows*). (*G*) Coronal post contrast T1-weighted image demonstrates heterogeneously enhancing intrasellar soft tissue. Subsequent biopsy revealed hemorrhagic infarction of a pituitary adenoma (*open arrow*).

frequently occur along the planum sphenoidale, along the clivus, at areas adjacent to the optic canal, and parasellar regions including the cavernous sinus. The symptomatic presentation related to mass effect of meningiomas in these areas will have considerable overlap with the presentation of pituitary tumors. Likewise, a variety of other lesions are known to have a predilection for the sellar and parasellar regions, including arachnoid cysts, Rathke cleft cysts, and craniopharyngiomas. Any of these lesions could potentially present during pregnancy as well.

Lymphocytic hypophysitis
Lymphocytic hypophysitis is an immune-mediated condition that most commonly occurs in women late in pregnancy or in the peripartum period; rare cases have been reported in men and children. The exact immune mechanism has not been elucidated and no reliable serologic assay exists, with biopsy required for definitive

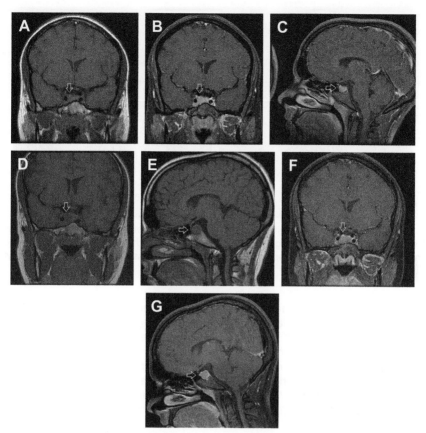

Fig. 15. A 23-year-old woman with known prolactinoma. (*A*) Precontrast and (*B, C*) postcontrast T1-weighted images demonstrate a lobulated, heterogeneously enhancing sellar mass with extension into the right cavernous sinus (*open arrow*). Eighteen weeks into her pregnancy, the patient presented with worsening headache and visual field disturbances. (*D, E*) Noncontrast T1-weighted images reveal marked interval enlargement of the macroadenoma with a convex superior margin and further cavernous sinus extension. (*F, G*) Postpartum, postcontrast T1-weighted images demonstrate reduction in macroadenoma size to near prepregnancy state.

diagnosis. Pathologically, lymphocytic infiltration of the adenohypophysis, neurohypophysis, and infundibular stalk occur, causing abnormal enlargement of the affected structures (**Fig. 16**). There is considerable overlap in the potential appearance of lymphocytic hypophysitis and a pituitary adenoma on MRI, both presenting as an enlarged pituitary mass. Certain imaging features may be helpful in distinguishing these entities, including timing of presentation, asymmetric enlargement of the gland (favors adenoma), thickening and enlargement of the hypothalamic stalk, and loss of the normal intrinsic T1 signal of the posterior pituitary (all favoring lymphocytic hypophysitis).[102] These imaging features are based on MR evaluation; evaluation of the pituitary stalk usually requires contrast administration for improved visualization.

Back Pain and Spinal Conditions

Primary spinal pathology

Back pain is a relatively common occurrence during pregnancy. Underlying causes range from relatively benign conditions such as hormone-related ligamentous laxity

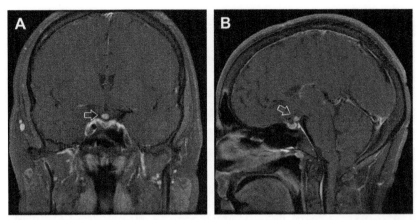

Fig. 16. A 34-year-old woman with hypothyroidism and diabetes insipidus. (*A*) Coronal and (*B*) sagittal postcontrast T1-weighted images demonstrate thickening and avid enhancement of the infundibulum (*open arrow*). Biopsy demonstrated marked lymphocytic infiltration.

and uterine compression of the lumbosacral plexus, to more serious conditions.[103,104] In the setting of trauma or a fall, CT may be used in cases of suspected fracture. CT likewise is often used as part of a trauma protocol for severe blunt injury. Otherwise, MRI should be the preferred method of evaluation, given the lack of ionizing radiation.

Acute intervertebral disc herniation is reported to occur in approximately 1 in 10,000 pregnancies, with progression to cauda equina syndrome being extremely rare among populations studied (**Fig. 17**).[105,106] As in nonpregnant populations, MRI is the preferred method of evaluation for any progressive neurologic syndrome.

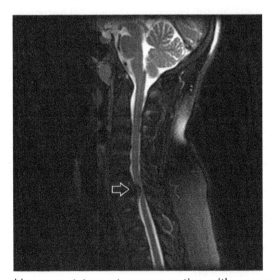

Fig. 17. A 28-year-old woman, status post cesarean section, with progressive neck and arm pain and lower extremity weakness. Sagittal T2-weighted image demonstrates severe spinal stenosis with cord compression at the C7-T1 level by a large disc protrusion/extrusion (*open arrow*).

Hormonally mediated acceleration of tumor growth could spur presentation of spinal meningiomas, as well as a variety of other lesions including spinal hemangiomas and giant cell tumors.[107–109] Imaging features of spinal meningiomas would include a discrete soft-tissue mass extrinsic to the spinal cord with a broad attachment at the dural surface. Spinal hemangiomas most frequently demonstrate elevated signal on both T1- and T2-weighted sequences, and often contain fat. Although these lesions demonstrate an elevated T2 signal, the presence of intralesional fat may result in a low-signal appearance if fat suppression is used. Spinal metastases related to gestational trophoblastic disease are also reported to cause progressive neurologic deficits.[99] Epidural hematomas may occur, which may be associated with pregnancy or be related to spinal and/or epidural anesthesia.[110,111] Likewise, epidural abscess formation may present spontaneously or be related to instrumentation.

With any progressive neurologic deficit, the key is to rule out a space-occupying lesion or involvement of the epidural space. Displacement or effacement of the T1

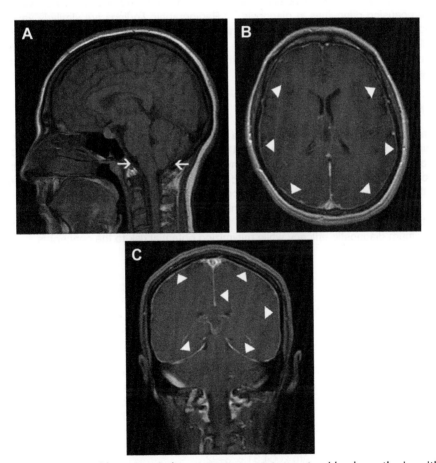

Fig. 18. A 33-year-old woman, 2 days postpartum, status post epidural anesthesia, with persistent headaches. (*A*) Sagittal T1-weighted image demonstrates mild descent of the brainstem and cerebellar tonsils with crowding at the foramen magnum (*small arrows*). (*B*) Axial and (*C*) coronal postcontrast T1-weighted images demonstrate mild, diffuse pachymeningeal thickening and enhancement (*arrowheads*).

bright epidural fat, displacement of the thecal sac dural margin, and narrowing of the thecal sac are all features of an epidural space abnormality. Abscesses may be heterogeneous in appearance or demonstrate elevated T2 signal, and may involve the epidural space circumferentially. The postcontrast appearance of epidural abscesses may demonstrate a combination of peripheral enhancement and diffuse enhancement, accounting for some element of phlegmon. Epidural hematomas tend to be intermediate or low signal on T1-weighted sequences acutely, and typically appear more focal and in the dorsal epidural space. Prompt recognition and diagnosis allows for rapid initiation of management.

Intracranial hypotension
Dural leaks of cerebrospinal fluid may occur following spinal interventions such as lumbar puncture, spinal surgery, or spinal anesthesia, or be related to epidural anesthesia with inadvertent dural puncture, possibly resulting in intracranial hypotension.[112,113] Clinically the hallmark presentation is that of positional headaches relieved in the recumbent position; however, symptoms and history may be varied, often causing difficulties in diagnosis.[114] Radiographic findings are similarly varied, and may include pachymeningeal enhancement, sagging of the brain, low-lying cerebellar tonsils, and subdural collections (**Fig. 18**).[115] In the postpartum patient with a history of spinal anesthesia, empiric therapy with an epidural blood patch may be used if conservative measures fail.

SUMMARY

In any pregnant patient presenting with a neurologic sign or symptom, it is important to consider both conditions directly related to pregnancy as well as those that may occur in any woman of reproductive age. Many of the conditions that could present during pregnancy frequently require diagnostic imaging as part of the workup. Recognition of the spectrum of imaging findings associated with the neurologic conditions of pregnancy allows for prompt diagnosis and initiation of therapy. With careful consideration, both CT and MRI may effectively be incorporated into evaluation algorithms for maximum diagnostic efficacy while minimizing potential risk to the conceptus.

REFERENCES

1. Hosley CM, McCullogh LD. Acute neurological issues in pregnancy and the peripartum. The Neurohospitalist 2011;1(2):104–16.
2. Royek AB, Parisi VM. Maternal biological adaptations to pregnancy. In: Hobbins JC, Reece EA, editors. Medicine of the fetus and mother. Philadelphia: Lippincott-Raven; 1999. p. 903–20.
3. Bentson J, Reza M, Winter J, et al. Steroids and apparent cerebral atrophy on computed tomography scans. J Comput Assist Tomogr 1978;2:16–23.
4. Oatridge A, Holdcroft A, Saeed N, et al. Change in brain size during and after pregnancy: study in healthy women and women with preeclampsia. AJNR Am J Neuroradiol 2002;23:19–26.
5. Foyouzi N, Yr Frisbaek BA, Norwitz ER. Pituitary gland and pregnancy. Obstet Gynceol Clin North Am 2004;31:873–92.
6. Karaca Z, Tanriverdi F, Unluhizarci K, et al. Pregnancy and pituitary disorders. Eur J Endocrinol 2010;162:453.
7. Dineen R, Banks A, Lenthall R. Imaging of acute neurological conditions in pregnancy and the puerperium. Clin Radiol 2005;60:1156.

8. Zak IT, Dulai HS, Kish KK. Imaging of neurologic disorders associated with pregnancy and postpartum period. Radiographics 2007;27:95.

9. Comeglio P, Fedi S, Liotta AA, et al. Blood clotting activation during normal pregnancy. Thromb Res 1996;84:199.

10. Kotsenas AL, Roth TC, Hershey BL, et al. Imaging neurologic complications of pregnancy and the puerperium. Acad Radiol 1999;6:243.

11. Martin JA, Hamilton BE, Ventura SJ, et al. Births: final data for 2009. Natl Vital Stat Rep 2011;60(1):1–70.

12. American Pregnancy.org. [Online] American Pregnancy Association. Cited: March 5, 2012. Available at: http://www.americanpregnancy.org/main/statistics. html. Accessed March 1, 2012.

13. American College of Radiology (ACR). ACR Guidelines and Technical Standards. ACR practice guideline for imaging pregnant or potentially pregnant adolescents and women with ionizing radiation. Reston (VA): American College of Radiology; 2008. p. 1–15.

14. American College of Radiology. ACR practice guideline for the use of intravascular contrast media. Reston (VA): American College of Radiology; 2007. p. 1–6.

15. European Society of Urogenital Radiology Contrast Media Safety Committee. ESUR guideline on contrast media: pregnancy and lactation. Vienna (Austria): European Society of Urogenital Radiology; 2008.

16. American College of Obstetricians and Gynecologists. Committee on Obstetric Practice. Guidelines for diagnostic imaging during pregnancy. Washington, DC: American College of Obstetricians and Gynecologists; 2004. reaffirmed 2009.

17. Wieseler KM, Bhargava P, Kanal KM, et al. Imaging in pregnant patients: examination appropriateness. Radiographics 2010;30:1215–33.

18. Goldberg-Stein SA, Liu B, Hahn PF, et al. Radiation dose management: part 2, estimating fetal radiation risk from CT during pregnancy. AJR Am J Roentgenol 2012;198:W352–6.

19. Swartz HM, Reichling BA. Hazards of radiation exposure for pregnant women. JAMA 1978;239:1907–8.

20. Saenger EI, Kereiakes JG. Medical radiation exposure during pregnancy. JAMA 1979;242(15):1669.

21. Mole RH. Childhood cancer after prenatal exposure to diagnostic X-ray examinations in Britain. Br J Cancer 1990;62:152–68.

22. Wakeford R, Little MP. Risk coefficients for childhood cancer after intrauterine irradiation. Int J Radiat Biol 2003;79(5):293–309.

23. Little MP. Leukaemia following childhood radiation exposure in the Japanese atomic bomb survivors and in medically exposed groups. Radiat Prot Dosimetry 2008;132(2):156–65.

24. Preston DL, Cullings H, Suyama A, et al. Solid cancer incidence in atomic bomb survivors exposed in utero or as young children. J Natl Cancer Inst 2008;100(6): 428–36.

25. Stewart A, Kneale GW. Radiation dose effects in relation to obstetric x-rays and childhood cancers. Lancet 1970;1(7658):1185–8.

26. Wagner LK, Lester RG, Saldana LR. Exposure of the pregnant patient to diagnostic radiations: a guide to medical management. Madison (WI): Medical Physics Publishing; 1997.

27. Hall EJ. Radiobiology of the radiologist. 4th edition. Chicago: Lippincott; 1984. p. 363–78, 419–52.

28. Berlin L. Radiation exposure and the pregnant patient. AJR Am J Roentgenol 1996;167:1377–9.

29. McCollough CH, Scheuler BA, Atwell TD, et al. Radiation exposure and pregnancy: when should we be concerned? Radiographics 2007;27:909–18.
30. Van Unnik JG, Broese JJ, Geleijns J, et al. Survey of CT techniques and absorbed dose in various Dutch hospitals. Br J Radiol 1997;70:367–71.
31. Huda W, Randazzo W, Tipnis S, et al. Embryo dose estimates in body CT. AJR Am J Roentgenol 2010;194:874–80.
32. Shetty MK. Abdominal computed tomography during pregnancy: a review of indications and fetal radiation exposure issues. Semin Ultrasound CT MR 2010;31:3–7.
33. Hurwitz LM, Yoshizumi T, Reiman RE, et al. Radiation dose to the fetus from body MDCT during early gestation. AJR Am J Roentgenol 2006;186:871–6.
34. Damilakis J, Perisinakis K, Voloudaki A, et al. Estimation of fetal radiation dose from computed tomography scanning in late pregnancy. Invest Radiol 2000; 35(9):527–33.
35. Angel E, Wellnitz CV, Goodsitt MM, et al. Radiation dose to the fetus for pregnant patients undergoing multidetector CT imaging: Monte Carlo simulations estimating fetal dose for a range of gestational age and patient size. Radiology 2008;249(1):220–7.
36. McCollough CH, Bruesewitz MR, Kofler JM. CT dose reduction and dose management tools: overview of available options. Radiographics 2006;26: 503–12.
37. Kaza RK, Platt JF, Al-Hawary MM, et al. CT enterography at 80 kVp with adaptive statistical iterative reconstruction versus at 120 kVp with standard reconstruction: image quality, diagnostic adequacy and dose reduction. AJR Am J Roentgenol 2012;198:1084–92.
38. Qi LP, Li Y, Tang L, et al. Evaluation of dose reduction and image quality in chest CT using adaptive statistical iterative reconstruction with the same group of patients. Br J Radiol 2012. [Epub ahead of print].
39. Desai GS, Uppot RN, Yu EW, et al. Impact of iterative reconstruction on image quality and radiation dose in multidetector CT of large body size adults. Eur Radiol 2012;22(8):1631–40.
40. Singh S, Kalra MK, Shenoy-Bhangle AS, et al. Radiation dose reduction with hybrid iterative reconstruction for pediatric CT. Radiology 2012;263(2): 537–46.
41. Lazarus E, DeBenedectis C, North D, et al. Utilization of imaging in pregnant patients: 10 year review of 5270 examinations in 3285 patients—1997-2006. Radiology 2009;251(2):517–24.
42. Helmrot E, Pettersson H, Sandborg M, et al. Estimation of dose to the unborn child at diagnostic x-ray examinations based on data registered in RIS/PACS. Eur Radiol 2007;17:205–9.
43. Kanal E, Barkovich AJ, Bell C, et al. ACR guidance document for safe MR practices 2007. AJR Am J Roentgenol 2007;188:1–27.
44. American College of Radiology - Society of Pediatric Radiology. ACR-SPR practice guideline for the safe and optimal performance of fetal magnetic resonance imaging (MRI). Reston (VA): American College of Radiology; 2010.
45. Gruters A, Krude H. Detection and treatment of congenital hypothyroidism. Nat Rev Endocrinol 2011;8(2):104–13.
46. Kriplani A, Relan S, Misra NK, et al. Ruptured intracranial aneurysm complicating pregnancy. Int J Gynaecol Obstet 1995;48:201.
47. Stoodley MA, Macdonald RL, Weir BK. Pregnancy and intracranial aneurysms. Neurosurg Clin N Am 1998;9:549.

48. Shah AK. Non-aneurysmal primary subarachnoid hemorrhage in pregnancy-induced hypertension and eclampsia. Neurology 2003;61:117.
49. Rother J, Waggie K, van Bruggen N, et al. Experimental cerebral venous thrombosis: evaluation using magnetic resonance imaging. J Cereb Blood Flow Metab 1996;16:1353–61.
50. Schaller B, Graf R, Sanada Y, et al. Hemodynamic changes after occlusion of the posterior superior sagittal sinus: and experimental PET study in cats. AJNR Am J Neuroradiol 2003;24:1876–80.
51. Yuh WT, Simonson TM, Wang AM, et al. Venous sinus occlusive disease: MR findings. AJNR Am J Neuroradiol 1994;15:309–16.
52. Leach JL, Fortuna RB, Jones BV, et al. Imaging of cerebral venous thrombosis: current techniques, spectrum of findings, and diagnostic pitfalls. Radiographics 2006;26:S19–41.
53. Wetzel SG, Kirsch E, Stock KW, et al. Cerebral veins: comparative study of CT venography in intraarterial digital subtraction angiography. AJNR Am J Neuroradiol 1999;20(2):249–55.
54. Renowden S. Cerebral venous sinus thrombosis. Eur Radiol 2004;14:215–26.
55. Simonds GR, Truwit CL. Anatomy of the cerebral vasculature. Neuroimaging Clin N Am 1994;4(4):691–706.
56. Alper F, Kantarci M, Dane S, et al. Importance of anatomical asymmetries of transverse sinuses: an MR venographic study. Cerebrovasc Dis 2004;18:236–9.
57. Casey SO, Ozsvath R, Choi JS. Prevalence of arachnoid granulation as detected with CT venography of the dural sinuses. AJNR Am J Neuroradiol 1997;18(5):993–4.
58. Strydom MA, Briers N, Bosman MC, et al. The anatomical basis of venographic filling defects of the transverse sinus. Clin Anat 2010;23(2):153–9.
59. White JB, Kaufman TJ, Kallmes DF. Venous sinus thrombosis: a misdiagnosis using MR angiography. Neurocrit Care 2008;8:290–2.
60. Zouaoui A, Hidden G. Cerebral venous sinuses: anatomical variants or thrombosis? Acta Anat (Basel) 1988;133:318–24.
61. Liang L, Korogi Y, Sugahara T, et al. Normal structures in the intracranial dural sinuses: delineation with 3D contrast enhanced magnetization prepared rapid acquisition gradient-echo imaging sequence. AJNR Am J Neuroradiol 2002; 23(10):1739–46.
62. Trimble CR, Harnsberger HR, Castillo M, et al. "Giant" arachnoid granulations just like CSF?: NOT!! AJNR Am J Neuroradiol 2010;31(9):1724–8.
63. Paavilainen T, Kurki T, Farkkila M, et al. Lower brain diffusivity in postpartum period compared to late pregnancy: results from a prospective imaging study of multiple sclerosis patients. Neuroradiology 2011. [Epub ahead of print].
64. Fox MW, Harms RW, Davis DH. Selected neurologic complications of pregnancy. Mayo Clin Proc 1990;65:1595.
65. Brass SD, Copen WA. Neurological disorders in pregnancy from a neuroimaging perspective. Semin Neurol 2007;27:411.
66. Linn J, Michl S, Katja B, et al. Cortical vein thrombosis; the diagnostic value of different imaging modalities. Neuroradiology 2010;52:899–911.
67. Favrole P, Guichard J, Crassard I, et al. Diffusion weighted imaging of intravascular clots in cerebral venous thrombosis. Stroke 2004;35:99–103.
68. Selim M, Fink J, Linfante I, et al. Diagnosis of cerebral venous thrombosis with echo-planar T2* weighted magnetic resonance imaging. Arch Neurol 2002;59:1021–6.
69. Isensee C, Reul J, Thron D. Magnetic resonance imaging of thrombosed dural sinuses. Stroke 1994;25:29–34.

70. Chu K, Kang DW, Yoon BW, et al. Diffusion weighted magnetic resonance in cerebral venous thrombosis. Arch Neurol 2001;58:1569–76.
71. Lovblad KO, Bassetti C, Schneider J, et al. Diffusion weighted MR in cerebral venous thrombosis. Cerebrovasc Dis 2001;11:169–76.
72. Ayanzen RH, Bird CR, Keller PJ, et al. Cerebral MR venography: normal anatomy, and potential diagnostic pitfalls. AJNR Am J Neuroradiol 2000; 21:74–8.
73. Gao K, Jiang H, Zhai JF, et al. Three-dimensional gadolinium enhanced MR venography to evaluate central venous steno-occlusive disease in hemodialysis patients. Clin Radiol 2012;30:1–4.
74. Lovblad KO, Schneider J, Bassetti C. Fast contrast enhanced MR whole-brain venography. Neuroradiology 2002;44:681–8.
75. Wetzel SG, Law M, Lee VL, et al. Imaging of the intracranial venous system with a contrast-enhanced volumetric interpolated examination. Eur Radiol 2003;13: 1010–8.
76. Kaplan PW, Repke JT. Eclampsia. Neurol Clin 1994;12:565.
77. Schwartz RB, Feske SK, Polak JF, et al. Preeclampsia-eclampsia: clinical and neuroradiographic correlates and insights into the pathogenesis of hypertensive encephalopathy. Radiology 2000;217:371.
78. Konstantinopoulous PA, Mousa S, Khairallah R, et al. Postpartum cerebral angiopathy: an important diagnostic consideration in the postpartum period. Am J Obstet Gynecol 2004;191:375.
79. Geocadin RG, Razumovsky AY, Wityk RJ, et al. Intracerebral hemorrhage and postpartum vasculopathy. J Neurol Sci 2002;205:29.
80. Chartier JP, Bousigue JY, Teisseyre A, et al. [Postpartum cerebral angiopathy of iatrogenic origin]. Rev Neurol (Paris) 1997;153:212 [in French].
81. Chiossi G, Neri I, Cavazzuti M, et al. Hyperemesis gravidarum complicated by Wernicke encephalopathy: background, case report, and review of the literature. Obstet Gynecol Surv 2006;61(4):255–68.
82. Kock-Henriksen N, Sorensen PS. The changing demographic pattern of multiple sclerosis epidemiology. Lancet Neurol 2010;9:520–32.
83. Confavreux C, Hutchinson M, Hours MM, et al. Rate of pregnancy related relapse in multiple sclerosis. N Engl J Med 1998;339:285–91.
84. Voskuhl RR, Gold SM. Sex-related factors in multiple sclerosis susceptibility and progression. Nat Rev Neurol 2012;8(5):255–63.
85. Whitacre CC, Reingold SC, O'Looney PA. A gender gap in autoimmunity. Science 1999;283:1277–8.
86. Vukusic S, Hutchinson M, Hours M, et al. For the pregnancy in multiple sclerosis group: pregnancy and multiple sclerosis (the PRIMS study): clinical predictors of postpartum relapse. Brain 2004;127:1353–60.
87. McDonald W, Compston A, Edan E, et al. Recommended diagnostic criteria for multiple sclerosis: guideline from the international panel on the diagnosis of multiple sclerosis. Ann Neurol 2001;50:121–7.
88. Polman CH, Reingold SC, Banwell B, et al. Diagnostic criteria for multiple sclerosis: 2010 revisions to the McDonald criteria. Ann Neurol 2011;69:292–302.
89. Miller DH, Grossman RI, Reingold SC, et al. The role of magnetic resonance techniques in understanding and managing multiple sclerosis. Brain 1998; 121:3–24.
90. Bruck W, Bitsch A, Kolenda H, et al. Inflammatory central nervous system demyelination: correlation of magnetic resonance imaging findings with lesion pathology. Ann Neurol 1997;42(5):783–93.

91. The EURAP Study Group. Seizure control and treatment in pregnancy. Observations from the EURAP epilepsy pregnancy registry. Neurology 2006;66:354–60.
92. Olafsson E, Hallgrimsson JT, Hauser WA, et al. Pregnancies of women with epilepsy: a population based study in Iceland. Epilepsia 1998;39:887–92.
93. Al Bunyan M, Abo-Talib Z. Outcome of pregnancies in epileptic women: a study in Saudi Arabia. Seizure 1999;8:26–9.
94. Fairgrieve SD, Jackson M, Jonas P, et al. Population based, prospective study of the care of women with epilepsy in pregnancy. Br Med J 2000;321:674–5.
95. Tomson T, Perucca E, Battino D. Navigating towards fetal and maternal health: the challenge of treating epilepsy in pregnancy. Epilepsia 2004;45(10):1171–5.
96. Harden CL, Meador KJ, Pennell PB, et al. Practice parameter update: management issues for women with epilepsy - focus on pregnancy (an evidence based review): teratogenesis and perinatal outcomes. Neurology 2009;73:133–41.
97. Vajda FJ. Treatment options for pregnant women with epilepsy. Expert Opin Pharmacother 2008;9(11):1859–68.
98. Altieri A, Franceschi S, Ferlay J, et al. Epidemiology and aetiology of gestational trophoblastic diseases. Lancet Oncol 2003;4:670–8.
99. Feng F, Xiang Y, Cao Y. Metastasis of gestational trophoblastic neoplasia to the spinal canal: a case report. J Reprod Med 2009;54(9):576–8.
100. Huang CY, Chen CA, Hsieh CY, et al. Intracerebral hemorrhage as initial presentation of gestational choriocarcinoma: a case report and literature review. Int J Gynecol Cancer 2007;17(5):1166–71.
101. Motivala S, Gologorsky Y, Kostandinov J, et al. Pituitary disorders during pregnancy. Endocrinol Metab Clin North Am 2011;40:827–36.
102. Gutenberg A, Larsen J, Lupi I, et al. A radiologic score to distinguish autoimmune hypophysitis from nonsecreting pituitary adenoma preoperatively. AJNR Am J Neuroradiol 2009;30:1766–72.
103. Chan YL, Lam WW, Lau TK, et al. Back pain in pregnancy: magnetic resonance imaging correlation. Clin Radiol 2002;57:1109–12.
104. Han I. Pregnancy and spinal problems. Curr Opin Obstet Gynecol 2010;22: 477–81.
105. LaBan MM, Perrin JC, Latimer FR. Pregnancy and the herniated lumbar disc. Arch Phys Med Rehabil 1983;64:319–21.
106. Mousavi SJ, Parnianpour M, Vleeming A, et al. Pregnancy related pelvic girdle pain and low back pain in an Iranian population. Spine 2007;32:E100–4.
107. Kiroglu Y, Benel B, Yagci B, et al. Spinal cord compression caused by vertebral hemangioma being symptomatic during pregnancy. Surg Neurol 2009;71: 487–92.
108. Kathiresan AS, Johnson JN, Hood BJ, et al. Giant cell tumor of the thoracic spine presenting in late pregnancy. Obstet Gynecol 2011;118:428–31.
109. Vijay K, Shetty AP, Rajasekaran S. Symptomatic vertebral hemangioma in pregnancy treated antepartum. A case report with review of literature. Eur Spine J 2008;17(Suppl 2):S299–303.
110. Case AS, Ramsey PS. Spontaneous epidural hematoma of the spine in pregnancy. Am J Obstet Gynecol 2005;193:875–7.
111. Loo CC, Dahlgren G, Irestedt L. Neurologic complications in obstetric regional anaesthesia. Int J Obstet Anesth 2000;9(2):99–124.
112. Bell WE, Joynt RJ, Sahs AL. Low spinal fluid pressure syndrome. Neurology 1960;10:512–21.
113. Rahman M, Bidari SS, Quisling RG, et al. Spontaneous intracranial hypotension: dilemmas in diagnosis. Neurosurgery 2011;69:4–14.

114. Schievink WI. Spontaneous spinal cerebrospinal fluid leaks and intracranial hypotension. JAMA 2006;295(19):2286–96.
115. Schievink WI, Maya MM, Louy C, et al. Diagnostic criteria for spontaneous spinal leaks and intracranial hypotension. AJNR Am J Neuroradiol 2008;29:853–6.

Neurologic Complications in the Patient Receiving Obstetric Anesthesia

Olajide Kowe, MBBS, FCARCSI*, Jonathan H. Waters, MD

KEYWORDS

• Neurology • Complications • Obstetric • Anesthesia

KEY POINTS

• Direct injury can result from failure to accurately determine the lower end of the spinal cord before needle placement.
• Peripheral nerve injury related to birth trauma is common but is frequently blamed on neuraxial anesthesia.
• Patients presenting with neuropathy caused by labor and delivery should be thoroughly examined and investigated.
• Nerve injuries secondary to birth trauma may take up to 10 weeks to resolve. Serial investigation such as nerve conduction studies may be needed to monitor recovery from the injury.

Neurologic deficits during or following labor and delivery often occur as a result of obstetric trauma. They can also be caused by neuraxial (epidural or spinal) anesthesia. Incidence of obstetric neuropathy has been estimated to be between 10 and 27 patients per 10,000 deliveries.[1] The true incidence of obstetric anesthesia neuropathy is unknown. Injury resulting from obstetric causes can occur in isolation or can present together with neuraxial anesthesia neurologic injury in the same patient. Obstetric factors that contribute to injuries during labor and delivery include instrumental delivery, short stature, prolonged labor, primiparous women, persistent transverse or posterior position of the fetal head, and prolonged lithotomy position in labor. Most of these injuries result from stretch or compression to a nerve. The most commonly injured nerve is the lateral femoral cutaneous nerve.[2] Epidural anesthesia

Financial support: None.
Department of Anesthesiology, Magee-Womens Hospital of University of Pittsburgh Medical Center, Pittsburgh, PA, USA
* Corresponding author. Department of Anesthesia, Yorkton Regional Hospital, 270 Bradbrooke Drive, SK S0A 2P0, Saskatchewan, Canada.
E-mail address: olajidekowe@gmail.com

has been associated with prolonged labor, which may contribute to neurologic injury from these obstetric causes.[3]

Anesthesia can also cause neurologic injury, although the mechanisms for these injuries are different from those of obstetric injury. Injury can result from direct trauma to the spinal cord, epidural hematoma, as well as other causes that are discussed in this article (**Table 1**). These injuries are less frequent than those of birth trauma, ranging from 0 to 12 per million women.[4]

ANESTHESIA-RELATED INJURY
Direct Spinal Cord Injury

Direct injury can result from failure to accurately determine the lower end of the spinal cord before needle placement. In approximately 80% of the adult population, the spinal cord ends at the level of the first lumbar vertebra, whereas the remaining 20% have spinal cords that extend to the level of the second lumbar vertebra.[5] As a result of this variation, placement of neuraxial block, especially spinal anesthesia, at a level below the second lumbar vertebra tends to reduce the incidence of direct spinal cord injury.[5,6]

Most trauma results from either direct catheter injury; direct needle injury to the spinal cord, spinal nerve roots, or conus medullaris; or intraneural injection of local anesthetics. Trauma to the spinal cord manifests as paresthesia or pain in the lower limbs that can be transient or persistent. If the patient experiences transient symptoms during the neuraxial block, the anesthesiologist may continue with the procedure, but if the paresthesia or pain persists in 1 or both limbs, then it is advisable to stop and reposition the needle or catheter. Local anesthetic injection into the epidural or intrathecal space should never be attempted in any patient who experiences persistent neurologic symptoms because sensory and motor block resulting from local anesthetics may mask the recognition of signs and symptoms of nerve injuries.

Table 1 Neuraxial-related injuries	
Injury Type	**Causes/Factors Implicated**
Spinal cord damage	
Direct injury	Unusually low conus medularis Traumatic catheterization High placement of needle
Indirect injury	Hematoma (epidural/spinal) Abscess (epidural/spinal)
Meningitis	
Infective	Bacterial, viral Aseptic
Noninfective	Chemical arachnoiditis
Spinal cord ischemia	Anterior spinal cord syndrome
Cauda equina syndrome	Intrathecal microcatheter Intrathecal lidocaine (high concentration)
Others	Dural puncture and cerebrospinal fluid leak (cranial nerve palsy) Total spinal block Back pain Seizures (systemic toxicity) Pneumocephalus

Epidural Hematoma

Epidural hematomas are rare but serious complications of neuraxial anesthesia. Incidence varies from 1:200,000 after spinal anesthesia to 1:150,000 after epidural placement.[7] Hematomas can occur in the presence of predisposing factors or without predisposing factors. Predisposing factors include gestational thrombocytopenia, preeclampsia/eclampsia, HELLP (hemolysis, elevated liver enzymes, and low platelet count) syndrome, and patients with inherited clotting dysfunctions. The most common anesthesia-related cause of epidural hematoma is placement of an epidural or spinal anesthetic in patients on anticoagulants or antiplatelet agents. Depending on the anticoagulant, it is important to delay neuraxial anesthesia until the effect of the drug has subsided (**Table 2**).[8] Patients with any predisposing factor should be investigated thoroughly before commencing with a neuraxial block. No patient should receive neuraxial anesthesia with full anticoagulation. It is important to carry out relevant laboratory investigations (for example, platelet counts, coagulation profile) in patients with risk factors.

The use of thromboelastography in patients at risk of bleeding has been recommended, if available, as an option to traditional laboratory testing.[9] The thromboelastograph (TEG) measures viscoelastic properties of clot formation and dissolution (platelet function, coagulation, fibrinogen-platelet interaction, and fibrinolysis). Obstetric patients often present with gestational thrombocytopenia, idiopathic thrombocytopenia, or thrombocytopenia associated with preeclampsia. In most of these patients, the TEG shows that these patients are hypercoagulable because of other changes in coagulation function caused by pregnancy. As a result, the TEG has shown that neuraxial block in patients with low platelet counts can be performed without complication.

Epidural hematoma should be suspected in patients showing any of the following symptoms: epidural anesthesia persisting for more than the expected duration of action of the local anesthetic used, unusual back pain and local tenderness, persistent numbness or motor weakness, or sphincter dysfunction. Quick diagnosis of an epidural hematoma is essential to prevent permanent neurologic injury. Urgent computed tomography (CT) scan or magnetic resonance imaging (MRI) is used to diagnose an epidural hematoma. Emergency surgical decompression within 6 hours of onset of signs and symptoms is necessary to avoid permanent damage.

Epidural Abscess

Epidural abscess is an uncommon complication of neuraxial techniques. Incidence in the general population varies from 1:1000 to 1:100,000 neuraxial blocks; however, in

Table 2	
Common anticoagulants and waiting periods before a neuraxial procedure	
Medication	**Before Neuraxial Procedure**
Unfractionated Heparin, low dose	No time restrictions
Unfractionated Heparin, high dose, intravenous, continuous	When activated partial thromboplastin time <40 s
Enoxaparin (Lovenox), low dose	12 h
Enoxaparin (Lovenox), high dose	24 h
Fondaparinux (Arixtra)	72 h
Clopidogrel (Plavix)	48 h
Eptifibatide (Integrelin)	8 h
Abciximab (Reopro)	48 h
Tirofiban (Aggrastat)	8 h

the obstetric population, it is much rarer, being estimated to occur in 1:500,000 epidural blocks.[10,11] It can occur spontaneously or after epidural block. Skin flora is usually the source of epidural abscess. *Staphylococcus aureus* is the commonest organism causing epidural abscess.[12] The risk of having an abscess increases with prolonged duration of epidural catheterization. As a result, most practitioners limit the duration of the catheter to 3 days. Other risk factors include patients with depressed immunity, and failure to adhere to aseptic conditions while performing neuraxial block. Clinical manifestation is similar to that of epidural hematoma. Clinical presentation includes fever, headache, back pain, malaise, and local tenderness. Nerve root pain develops within 3 to 5 days of the onset of back pain and this leads gradually to leg weakness, paraplegia, and bladder or bowel dysfunction. Urgent CT scan or MRI with gadolinium should be done to confirm the diagnosis of epidural abscess. Aggressive antimicrobial therapy is the mainstay of treatment of epidural abscess. Surgical decompression is necessary if there are features of nerve root compression.

Meningitis

This is a rare complication of neuraxial block. The incidence has been estimated to be around 1:39,000 neuraxial procedures.[13] Incidence decreases with procedures done under strict aseptic conditions (facemask, sterile gloves, and cap). Microbial contamination from the mouth and nose are the commonest cause of meningitis after epidural or subarachnoid block. Most meningitis resulting from neuraxial procedures are caused by *Streptococcus viridans*. Clinical manifestations of meningitis are similar to those of postdural puncture headache. Features include fever, malaise, headache, irritability, altered consciousness level, neck stiffness, and Kerning or Brudzinski signs. Management of meningitis involves a thorough physical examination, laboratory investigation, and aggressive antimicrobial therapy. Complete blood count, cerebrospinal fluid (CSF) analysis, and blood culture should be done. Laboratory investigation must not delay commencement of antimicrobial therapy because this is the mainstay of treatment.

Chemical meningitis (arachnoiditis) can also complicate epidural or spinal anesthesia. It occurs as a result of accidental injection of contaminated local anesthetics into the subarachnoid or epidural space. Chemical arachnoiditis can also result from traces of chlorhexidine containing skin preparations being transmitted into the subarachnoid space on a needle used for a neuraxial procedure. Clinical features are difficult to differentiate from infective meningitis. It is a diagnosis of exclusion. Although chemical meningitis resolves spontaneously, aggressive antimicrobial therapy is advised because of problems in differentiating this condition from meningitis caused by microbes.

Anterior Spinal Artery Syndrome (Cord Ischemia)

This syndrome is extremely rare in obstetric anesthesia. The anterior two-thirds of the spinal cord is supplied by the anterior spinal artery. This region is reinforced by radicular arteries originating from the thoracolumbar aorta, the largest of which is the artery of Adamkiewicz. Anterior spinal artery syndrome is often associated with severe, prolonged hypotension, arteriosclerosis, or surgery that interferes with blood flow to the arteries.[14] There has been a suggestion that epinephrine-containing local anesthetics may also predispose patients with vascular disease to this phenomenon.[15] The most common causes for this syndrome relate to major spine instrumentation and thoracolumbar aneurysm repair.[16] This condition manifests as paraplegia, loss of pain and temperature sensation, and bladder and bowel incontinence. Sensations of proprioception, light touch, and vibration are all spared in this syndrome because they involve the posterior spinal column. Cord ischemia is diagnosed using diffusion-weighted MRI because diagnosis using convectional MRI is difficult in early stage of acute cord ischemia.

Cauda Equina Syndrome

This syndrome has been described after the use of lidocaine for spinal anesthesia. In the early 1990s, continuous intrathecal microcatheters were introduced. Shortly thereafter, reports of cauda equine syndrome were made.[17,18] This was initially associated with the microcatheter; however, subsequent investigation revealed that pooling of local anesthetic, most specifically lidocaine, was the causative agent. Lidocaine and, to some extent, tetracaine, have the greatest potential to cause neurotoxicity. Patients with diabetic neuropathy tend to be prone to this toxicity.

Cauda equina syndrome is a dysfunction of nerve roots L2 to S5. It manifest as burning low back pain, sphincter dysfunction, paraplegia, and sensory dysfunction in the perineum (saddle anesthesia). Although not as severe as cauda equine syndrome, transient neurotoxicity associated with lidocaine spinal anesthesia has been reported.[19] This transient neurotoxicity presents as back pain that can last several days following an anesthetic. As a result, few conscientious practitioners use lidocaine when performing spinal anesthesia.

Postdural Puncture Headache

Postdural puncture headache (PDPH) can occur after epidural with recognized or unrecognized dural puncture. It can also occur after subarachnoid block. PDPH after epidural most often results from needle puncture of the dural sac or during catheter placement. Headache is caused by continuous CSF leak through the hole in the dural sac and continuous traction on the meninges and meningeal vessels.[20] Symptoms usually occur 24 to 48 hours after dural puncture, although they may occur shortly after dural puncture. Headache resulting from CSF leak is bilateral, fronto-occipital, radiates to the neck, and worsens on standing or sitting upright. The headache is relieved by lying supine. Other symptoms include photophobia, neck stiffness, and nausea. Diplopia and tinnitus may be experienced secondary to traction on the sixth cranial nerve. Incidence of PDPH depends on the size of the needle and the nature of the tip of the needle.[21] In general, using a small-gauge needle with a pencil point reduces the incidence of PDPH. The incidence of PDPH is also higher with patients less than 45 years of age and also with pregnant patients.[20] It is important to differentiate PDPH from meningitis, because the latter is associated with fever and increased white blood cells count.

Treatment of PDPH includes conservative management or blood patch. Conservative management involves bed rest for patients who do not tolerate ambulation, adequate rehydration, and analgesics. Intravenous (IV) or oral caffeine has been advocated to speed CSF production.[22] Other conservative management that has been tried includes sumatriptan,[23] adrenocorticotropic hormone, theophylline,[24] and use of an abdominal binder. Epidural blood patch should be done for patients who do not respond to conservative management or who manifest neurologic symptoms like diplopia or tinnitus. Diplopia or tinnitus can be permanent, so a prompt blood patch is indicated in this subset of patients.

A blood patch done less than 24 hours after the dural puncture has a high failure rate (about 75% failure rate). In some circumstances, following a dural puncture, the anesthesiologist places an epidural catheter. Some have advocated that, following delivery, a prophylactic blood patch be performed in advance of symptoms. However, prophylactic blood patch has a high failure rate.

Before performing a blood patch, it is important to make sure that the patient is not septic and does not have preeclampsia or other causes for headache. This procedure involves injection of 20 mL of autologous blood into the epidural space. Injection of blood should be stopped if the patient experiences back pain or neurologic symptoms in the lower limbs.[25] Epidural blood patch should be performed under strict aseptic conditions. The patient must be informed that the risk of performing a blood patch is same as placement of the original neuraxial block. It is advisable to do an epidural blood patch at a level lower than initial neuraxial block because 70% of the injected blood will spread cephalad. An epidural blood patch performed later than 24 hours after wet tap has success rate of 70% to 97%.[26] If 2 epidural blood patches have been performed, and the patient still complains of a headache, then other causes for the headache should be sought.

Total Spinal Block

When performing an epidural block, the epidural catheter is sometimes accidentally threaded into the subarachnoid space. To test for this complication, a test dose of local anesthetic is given. This test dose involves a small amount of local anesthetic that results in a spinal block if the catheter is in the subarachnoid space. When the test dose is not performed, or inadequate time expires between the test dose and the regular epidural dose, a total spinal block can occur. A total spinal block results when a large volume of local anesthetic, intended for the epidural space, is injected into the subarachnoid space, which can result in anesthesia of the spinal cord, cervical spinal nerves, and brainstem. The incidence of total spinal block is unknown.

When a total spinal block occurs, the symptoms are typically severe. First, patients mention that their lower extremities are paralyzed, followed by complaints of the inability to breath. Respiratory arrest follows shortly thereafter. Cardiovascular collapse follows with profound hypotension and bradycardia.

Management of a total spinal block is mainly supportive. A high index of suspicion is important in early diagnosis and also in preventing irreversible organ damage in patients with total spinal block. Quick recognition of this condition is important in preventing irreversible organ damage and death of the fetus. Reverse Trendelenburg may help to limit further cranial spread of local anesthetics. Management is targeted toward symptoms and organ systems. For the cardiovascular system, hypotension should be treated with vasopressors/inotropes (eg, ephedrine, phenylephrine, epinephrine, or norepinephrine). Bradycardia can be treated with atropine or glycopyrrolate. Respiratory collapse should be managed with 100% oxygen, positive pressure ventilation, and intubation.

A total spinal block results from an excessive amount of local anesthetic being injected into the subarachnoid space. There are several factors that may predispose a patient to a total spinal block. First, obese patients tend to have a reduced subarachnoid space, which may favor cephalad spread of local anesthetics. Obesity also increases intra-abdominal pressure and may increase risk of high block. Pregnancy may also favor cephalad spread of local anesthetic in the subarachnoid space secondary to increased intra-abdominal pressure. Fluid or local anesthetic in the epidural space may compress the subarachnoid space, which may predispose such patients to total spinal block if they subsequently have a subarachnoid block. This condition typically occurs when an epidural has been deemed inadequate to perform a cesarean section.

Pharmacology of the local anesthetic can also influence spread of the drug. For instance, the baricity of the drug affects the spread. Baricity is the specific gravity of the drug relative to the CSF. Hyperbaric drugs sink in the subarachnoid space because the heavier drug displaces the lighter CSF. Hypobaric drugs rise in the subarachnoid space. Most local anesthetics used for spinal anesthesia are in the hyperbaric category. Local anesthetics used for epidural anesthesia are isobaric; their density is similar to that of CSF, so they tend to stay in the location of their injection. The spread of local anesthetic can be controlled by manipulating patient position. The dose and volume of local anesthetic also determine the level of the block.

Back Pain

Although back pain is a common complication of neuraxial block, most obstetric patients have some degree of back pain following delivery, regardless of whether they had a neuraxial block. The incidence of anesthesia-related back pain varies from 15% for spinal anesthesia to 30% for epidural anesthesia. Pain secondary to neuraxial block is mostly self-limiting. Pain may be an early feature of serious complications of neuraxial block such as epidural/subarachnoid hematoma or an abscess. Therefore, patients complaining of unusual back pain after neuraxial anesthesia should be thoroughly investigated.

Factors contributing to development of back pain after neuraxial anesthesia include multiple attempts/traumatic manipulation, ligamentous injury, periosteal trauma, and local inflammation. Management of postneuraxial anesthesia back pain is conservative and most cases resolve within a few days to a few weeks. Reassurance is all that is needed after excluding serious complications that might present with back pain. Analgesics like nonsteroidal antiinflammatory drugs and acetaminophen can be prescribed for severe and prolonged back pain. Back pain after neuraxial anesthesia can persist as chronic back pain.

Seizure from Systemic Toxicity of Local Anesthetics

This complication occurs after inadvertent intravascular injection of local anesthetic. It is extremely rare after spinal anesthesia because of the small volume/dose of local anesthetic required to achieve a good surgical block. Systemic toxicity can occur after obstetric epidural anesthesia or caudal block because larger volumes of local anesthetics are used for both procedures.[27] Toxicity mostly affects the central nervous system and the cardiovascular system. Factors affecting patient response to inadvertent intravascular injection of local anesthetic include the type of local anesthetic used. Bupivacaine is the most toxic, followed (in order of decreasing toxicity) by ropivacaine, levobupivacaine, lidocaine, and chloroprocaine. The rate of the injection dictates the peak serum level, so a faster injection results in a quicker onset of systemic toxicity.

Local anesthetics act as membrane stabilizers by binding to sodium channels. The duration of the binding varies among different drugs. Bupivacaine binds almost irreversibly to sodium channels and thus has the highest toxicity of all the local anesthetics. Therefore, they alter the electrical activities of excitable tissues such as the neurons and cardiac muscles. The end result is central nervous system and cardiovascular system depression. Early signs and symptoms of systemic toxicity include agitation, metallic taste in the mouth, circumoral paresthesia, diplopia, tinnitus, and confusion. Late signs include seizures caused by inhibition of inhibitory neurons in the central nervous system, and loss of consciousness. Further neurologic deterioration can result in cardiovascular collapse with hypotension, arrhythmias, and cardiac arrest.

It is important to use preventive measures when administering local anesthetic drugs into the epidural space. Such techniques include aspiration of the epidural catheter before giving a dose to exclude an intravascular catheter; dosing the epidural catheter with incremental doses of the drug, rather than single large dose; and the use of local anesthetic containing epinephrine, which can help to detect intravascular catheters because patients will experience tachycardia.

Early recognition of signs and symptoms of systemic toxicity helps to institute early management and thus may prevent death. Hospitals administering neuraxial blocks for obstetric patients should have facilities for managing toxicity resulting from local anesthetics. Lipid emulsion is the mainstay of treatment of local anesthetic toxicity.[28] A 20% intralipid should be given first because a 1.5-mL/kg IV bolus dose given over 60 seconds followed by a 0.25-mL/kg/min IV (400 mL) infusion over 30 to 40 minutes. The infusion of lipid should be maintained until a stable cardiovascular system exists. Cardiopulmonary bypass should be requested if available. It is important to continue cardiopulmonary resuscitation during lipid emulsion administration. Recovery from local anesthetic toxicity may take up to 2 hours.

Pneumocephalus

This condition is also referred to as intracerebral pneumatocele or aerocele. Pneumo-cephalus occurs when there is gas within the intracranial cavity (intraparenchymal, subarachnoid, intraventricular, epidural, and subdural). Pneumocephalus can occur after epidural anesthesia, caudal block, and spinal anesthesia.[29] The epidural space is typically identified by a technique called loss of resistance. An epidural needle is placed through the skin and subcutaneous fat, into one of the spinal ligaments. As the needle is advanced from the ligamentum flavum into the epidural space, a syringe containing air or saline is placed onto the needle. Pressure is applied on the barrel of the syringe as the needle is advanced. When the epidural space is entered, the air or saline is easily injected; while passing through the ligaments, it is not. If the epidural space is missed and the subarachnoid space is entered instead, the air or saline is injected into the CSF. Pneumocephalus is especially prominent with the use of air to find the loss of resistance; however, saline is never free of air when it is used. It has also been described after subarachnoid block.

Pneumocephalus presents with clinical features similar to those of postdural puncture headache, meningitis, and chemical arachnoiditis. Therefore, this condition should be considered in any obstetric patient presenting with features that suggest meningitis without fever or persistent headache after treatment of postdural puncture headache with blood patch. A pneumocephalus behaves like a space-occupying lesion in the rigid cranium and thus manifests signs and symptoms of raised intracra-nial pressure. Clinical manifestations of pneumocephalus include nausea, vomiting, headache, blurring of vision, tinnitus, dizziness, seizures, and may result in a depressed level of consciousness. These manifestations are rare following an epidural block but have been reported from pneumocephalus caused by a neurosur-gical procedure or head and face trauma.

Diagnosis of intracranial aerocele can be made using CT scan of the brain, which shows characteristic multiple small air bubbles in the cistern compressing the frontal lobe (Mount Fuji sign). This condition can also be diagnosed using plain radiograph. Management of pneumocephalus after obstetric neuraxial anesthesia is mainly conservative and involves patient reassurance, bed rest, and analgesics (acetamino-phen, opioids, nonsteroidal antiinflammatory drugs).

OBSTETRIC BIRTH TRAUMA

Peripheral nerve injury related to birth trauma is common but is frequently blamed on neuraxial anesthesia. For this reason, it is important for the neurologist to understand the mechanism and presentation of these injuries (**Table 3**).

Table 3 Obstetric palsies	
Obstetric Palsy	**Manifestations**
Lumbosacral trunk	Quadriceps and hip adductor weakness, foot drop
Lateral femoral cutaneous nerve	Numbness on anterolateral thigh
Common peroneal nerve	Paresthesia on lateral calf and foot drop
Femoral nerve	Paresthesia of the thigh and calf, weak hip flexion, and weakness of quadriceps muscles
Obturator nerve	Paresthesia on medial side of the thigh and weakness of hip adduction

Lumbosacral Plexus Nerve Injury

The lumbosacral plexus originates from nerve roots L4 to S5. Injury to the plexus can occur by compression of the fetal head against the posterior rim of the pelvic bone, especially with forceps delivery. Injury to the L4 to S5 plexus can be unilateral (75%) or bilateral (25%). Lumbosacral plexus injury affects the quadriceps and hip adductors and manifests as foot drop.

Lateral Femoral Cutaneous Nerve Injury

This nerve originates from nerve root L2 to L3 and passes beneath the inguinal ligament to innervate the anterior thigh (sensory). It can be compressed during prolonged pushing in the lithotomy position or stirrups position. Injury to the lateral femoral cutaneous nerve manifests as numbness of the anterolateral thigh, also known as meralgia paresthetica.

Common Peroneal Nerve Injury

The common peroneal nerve originates from nerve roots L4 to S2. This nerve can be injured as it winds around the head of the fibula, where compression can occur especially in prolong lithotomy or stirrups position. It manifest as paresthesia in the lateral calf and foot drop.

Femoral Nerve Injury

The femoral nerve originates from the L2 to L4 nerve roots. It can be compressed along its route as it passes beneath the inguinal ligament lateral to the femoral artery, which happens during prolong pushing with the hip excessively flexed. It manifest as paresthesia of the thigh and calf, weak hip flexion, and weakness of quadriceps muscles.

Obturator Nerve Injury

The obturator nerve originates from nerve roots L2 to L4 and passes through the obturator canal on the lateral pelvic wall, where compression can occur by the fetal head or during forceps delivery. Injury to this nerve manifests as paresthesia in the medial side of the thigh and weakness of hip adduction.

DIAGNOSIS AND MANAGEMENT OF BIRTH TRAUMA–RELATED NEUROPATHY

Patients presenting with neuropathy caused by labor and delivery should be thoroughly examined and investigated. The following questions help in detecting the cause of the injury:

- What was the timing of onset of symptoms?
- What is the location and severity of the symptoms?
- Are the symptoms progressing or regressing?
- Do they radiate?
- Did the patient receive neuraxial anesthesia?
- Was there any paresthesia elicited during placement of the neuraxial needle?
- If a paresthesia was elicited, what was its duration? Was it persistent or transient?
- Did the patient have full recovery from neuraxial anesthesia after delivery?
- What was the duration of labor?
- What was the position assumed by the patient during pushing, and for how long?
- Was any instrumentation used for the delivery (eg, forceps)?

Any significant finding in such patient should be documented. Investigations that can help in diagnosing such injury include MRI, CT, electromyography, and nerve conduction studies. Nerve injuries secondary to birth trauma may take up to 10 weeks to resolve. Serial investigation (eg, nerve conduction studies) may be needed to monitor recovery from the injury.

REFERENCES

1. Wong CA, Scavone BM, Dugan S, et al. Incidence of post partum lumbosacral spine and lower extremity nerve injuries. Obstet Gynecol 2003;101:279–88.
2. Dar AQ, Robinson APC, Lyons G. Postpartum neurologic symptoms following regional blockade: a prospective study with case controls. Int J Obstet Anesth 2002;11:85–90.
3. Alexander JM, Lucas MJ, Ramin SM, et al. The course of labor with and without epidural analgesia. Am J Obstet Gynecol 1998;178:516–20.
4. Ruppen W, Derry S, McQuay H, et al. Incidence of epidural hematoma, infection, and neurologic injury in obstetric patients with epidural analgesia/anesthesia. Anesthesiology 2006;105:394–9.
5. Broadbent CR, Maxwell WB, Ferrie R, et al. Ability of anaesthetists to identify a marked lumbar interspace. Anaesthesia 2000;55:1122–6.
6. Fettes PD, Wildsmith JA. Somebody else's nervous system. Br J Anaesth 2002; 88:760–3.
7. Brooks H, May A. Neurological complications following regional anesthesia in obstetrics. British Journal of Anaesthesia 2003;3:111–4.
8. Horlocker TT, Wedel DJ, Rowlingson JC, et al. Regional anesthesia in the patient receiving antithrombotic or thrombolytic therapy: American Society of Regional Anesthesia and Pain Medicine evidence-based guidelines (third edition). Reg Anesth Pain Med 2010;35:64–101.
9. Bigeleisen PE, Kang Y. Thrombelastography as an aid to regional anesthesia: preliminary communication. Reg Anesth 1991;16:59–61.
10. Moen V, Dahlgren N, Irestedt L. Severe neurologic complications after central neuraxial blockades in Sweden 1990-1999. Anesthesiology 2004;101:950–9.
11. Scott DB, Hibbard BM. Serious non-fatal complications associated with extradural block in obstetric practice. Br J Anaesth 1990;64:537–41.
12. Grewal S, Hocking G, Wildsmith JA. Epidural abscesses. Br J Anaesth 2006;96: 292–302.
13. Reynolds F. Neurological infections after neuraxial anesthesia. Anesthesiol Clin 2008;26:23–52.

14. Eastwood DW. Anterior spinal artery syndrome after epidural anesthesia in a pregnant diabetic patient with scleroderma. Anesth Analg 1991;73:90–1.
15. Tetzlaff JE, Dilger J, Yap E, et al. Cauda equina syndrome after spinal anaesthesia in a patient with severe vascular disease. Can J Anaesth 1998;45:667–9.
16. Zuber WF, Gaspar MR, Rothschild PD. The anterior spinal artery syndrome–a complication of abdominal aortic surgery: report of five cases and review of the literature. Ann Surg 1970;172(5):909–15.
17. Rigler ML, Drasner K, Krejcie TC, et al. Cauda equina syndrome after continuous spinal anesthesia. Anesth Analg 1991;72:275–81.
18. Schell RM, Brauer FS, Cole DJ, et al. Persistent sacral nerve root deficits after continuous spinal anaesthesia. Can J Anaesth 1991;38:908–11.
19. Schneider M, Ettlin T, Kaufmann M, et al. Transient neurologic toxicity after hyperbaric subarachnoid anesthesia with 5% lidocaine. Anesth Analg 1993;76:1154–7.
20. Turnbull DK, Shepherd DB. Post-dural puncture headache: pathogenesis, prevention and treatment. Br J Anaesth 2003;91:718–29.
21. Reynolds F. Damage to conus medularis after spinal anesthesia (case report). Anaesthesia 2001;56:238–47.
22. Camann WR, Murray RS, Mushlin PS, et al. Effects of oral caffeine on postdural puncture headache. A double-blind, placebo-controlled trial. Anesth Analg 1990;70:181–4.
23. Carp H, Singh PJ, Vadhera R, et al. Effects of the serotonin receptor agonist sumatriptan on postdural puncture headache: report of six cases. Anesth Analg 1994;79:180–2.
24. Schwalbe SS, Schiffmiller MW, Marx GF. Theophylline for post-dural puncture headache [abstract]. Anesthesiology 1991;75:A1082.
25. Abouleish E, Vega S, Blendinger I, et al. Long term follow up of epidural blood patch. Anesth Analg 1975;54:459–63.
26. Crawford JS. Experiences with epidural blood patch. Anaesthesia 1980;35:513–5.
27. Dillane D, Finucane BT. Local anesthetic systemic toxicity. Can J Anaesth 2010;57:368–80.
28. Brull SJ. Lipid emulsion for the treatment of local anesthetic toxicity: patient safety implications. Anesth Analg 2008;106:1337–9.
29. Roderick L, More DC, Artru AA. Pneumocephalus with headache during spinal anesthesia. Anesthesiology 1985;62:690–2.

Headache in Pregnancy

E. Anne MacGregor, MB BS, MD, MFSRH, MICR[a,b,*]

KEYWORDS

- Migraine • Menstrual migraine • Pregnancy • Headache • Eclampsia

KEY POINTS

- Most headaches follow a benign course during pregnancy.
- Hypertensive disorders of pregnancy and stroke are more likely to occur in women with a history of migraine.
- Management of headaches during pregnancy is essentially similar to management during the nonpregnant state.
- Women benefit from early advice on drugs that can be continued during pregnancy.

INTRODUCTION

Most people have headaches at some point during their lives. The common primary headaches, tension-type headache and migraine, are predominantly a female affliction, particularly during childbearing years. A review of global population-based data identified a lifetime prevalence of tension-type headache in 49% of women and 42% of men, and a lifetime prevalence of migraine in 22% of women and 10% of men.[1] Trigeminal autonomic cephalalgias are rare, affecting less than 1 per 1000 of the population.[2] Whereas paroxysmal hemicrania has a 2.1 to 2.4:1 female to male ratio, cluster headache is predominantly a male disorder (female to male ratio 1:2.5–7.5) but is often undiagnosed in women.[2,3]

Although primary headaches typically improve during pregnancy, some women experience more frequent and severe headaches while a few develop headache for the first time. Primary headaches do not in themselves pose any threat to pregnancy, but migraine is associated with increased risk of hypertensive disorders of pregnancy. Frequent prepregnancy headache is a strong predictor of poor general and emotional

The author has acted as a paid consultant to, and/or her department has received research funding from Addex, Allergan, AstraZeneca, Bayer Healthcare, Berlin-Chemie, BTG, Endo Pharmaceuticals, GlaxoSmithKline, Menarini, Merck, Pozen and Unipath. She received no financial support for the preparation of this article.

[a] Barts Sexual Health Centre, St Bartholomew's Hospital, London EC1A 7BE, UK; [b] Centre for Neuroscience and Trauma, Blizard Institute of Cell and Molecular Science, Barts and the London School of Medicine and Dentistry, London E1 1AT, UK
* Barts Sexual Health Centre, St Bartholomew's Hospital, London EC1A 7BE.
E-mail address: e.macgregor@qmul.ac.uk

Neurol Clin 30 (2012) 835–866
doi:10.1016/j.ncl.2012.04.001
0733-8619/12/$ – see front matter © 2012 Elsevier Inc. All rights reserved.

neurologic.theclinics.com

health during pregnancy and should alert the health care professional to assess these women for depressive disorders.[4] Drug treatment is usually necessary for control of severe headaches, so health care providers need to advise women on safe and effective treatment during pregnancy and lactation. Of more concern is that approximately half of the pregnancies in the United States are unplanned, of which more than 40% continue to birth.[5] Hence health care providers need accurate knowledge of the likely effects of inadvertent drug use on the outcome of the pregnancy.

EFFECT OF PREGNANCY AND LACTATION ON PRIMARY HEADACHES
Tension-Type Headache

Despite being more prevalent than migraine, there are few studies assessing the effect of pregnancy on tension-type headache. In a retrospective cross-sectional population-based study of 102 women with tension-type headache, 28% reported improvement during pregnancy, 67% reported no change, and 5% reported increased headache.[6] In a study of 33 women with tension-type headache completing a questionnaire 3 days postpartum, 82% reported improvement during pregnancy (49% complete remission) and 18% reported no change.[7] In a prospective cohort study of 856 women diagnosed with nonmigraine headache prepregnancy, 25.1% had complete remission during pregnancy.[8]

In the population-based Nord-Trøndelag Health Study in Norway from 1995 to 1997, 9281 women were 40 years or younger and responded to questions on headache, pregnancy, and birth, of whom 550 were pregnant at the time of completing the questionnaire.[9] Adjusting for age and educational level, the nonmigraine 1-year prevalence was lower in pregnant than in nonpregnant women. The association between headache and pregnancy was significant for women pregnant with their first child (odds ratio [OR] 0.6, 95% confidence interval [CI] 0.4–0.8), but not for multiparous women (OR 0.9, 95% CI 0.7–1.1). Of 20,287 nonpregnant women who were 70 years or younger, women without children tended to have fewer nonmigraine headaches in comparison with women with children, although the difference was not significant (OR 1.1, 95% CI 1.0–1.2).

Cluster Headache

Because cluster headache is relatively rare and more prevalent in men, data on the effect of pregnancy is limited. In a study of 34 women with cluster headache, 8 had had 13 pregnancies since the onset of cluster headache, of whom 6 were completely free or almost free from headache during all 9 of their pregnancies.[10] Two women experienced cluster headache during 4 pregnancies. In addition, 3 women were followed during and after pregnancy. The first experienced a single attack during pregnancy, a moderately severe attack 3 days after delivery, and a severe attack 3 weeks later, followed by a typical cluster lasting for 6 weeks at 5 months postpartum. The second had a period of cluster headache starting 1 and 3 days, respectively, after 2 deliveries. The third woman experienced cluster headache starting 3 days after delivery.

In a questionnaire study of 65 women with cluster headache recruited from a specialist clinic, 58 reported symptoms during their reproductive years.[3] Of these, 3 women experienced cluster-headache attacks during pregnancy and 3 reported that an expected cluster period did not occur during pregnancy. One woman experienced cluster headache after birth on 2 occasions.

In a population-based questionnaire study of 143 women with cluster headaches, 53 had their first attack before their first pregnancy, 89 had their first attack after their first pregnancy, and 1 woman experienced her first attack during her first pregnancy.[11] Of 19 (17%) women who experienced cluster headache during a pregnancy, 11 reported no increase in severity or frequency during pregnancy compared with attacks outside pregnancy, 3 reported improvement, and 5 reported increased attack frequency and/or severity. Twenty-six women (23%) reported that they missed an expected cluster period during pregnancy, of whom 8 experienced a cluster period within 1 month postpartum.

It has been noted that women who have their first cluster headache before their first pregnancy have fewer children than those who already have children at the time of their first attack.[10,11] Although the possibility of hypofertility has been raised, the more likely explanation is that women choose not to conceive because they are concerned about the effects of medication for cluster headache on the outcome of pregnancy.[11]

Migraine

Migraine is particularly affected by hormonal fluctuations. In menstruating women, declining estrogen after period of stable levels is associated with increased risk of migraine without aura.[12,13] By contrast, high plasma concentrations of estrogen are associated with attacks of migraine with aura.[14] It could be predicted that high, stable levels of placental estrogen during the pregnancy should benefit migraine without aura but not migraine with aura.

In line with this hypothesis, retrospective and prospective studies suggest that around 60% to 70% of migraineurs experience improvement in migraine during pregnancy; in around 20% attacks completely disappear (**Fig. 1, Tables 1–3**).[7,8,15–32] If no improvement is seen toward the end of the first trimester, migraine is likely to continue throughout pregnancy and postpartum.[31] Improvement is more likely in women with a history of menstrual rather than nonmenstrual headaches (**Fig. 2**) and in women with a prepregnancy history of migraine without aura rather than migraine with aura (**Fig. 3**).[7,15,18–23,26,32]

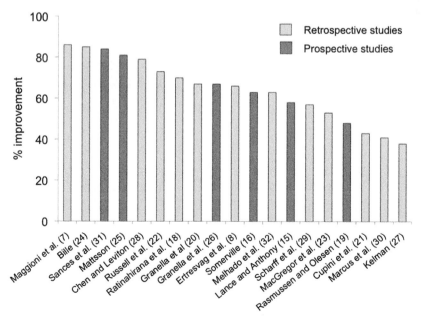

Fig. 1. Percentage of women reporting improvement of migraine during pregnancy.

Table 1
Retrospective studies of the effect of pregnancy on migraine

Study	Sample Size	Outcome			
		Improved (%)	No Change (%)	Increased (%)	New Onset (%)
Lance and Anthony[15]	120	58	42		NA
Somerville[16]	38	63 (19 complete remission)	19		19
Manzoni et al[17]	74: 36 MO, 38 MA	NR	16 MO / 40 MA (P<.05)		3 MO / 26 MA (P<.05)
Ratinahirana et al[18]	116: 90 MO, 26 MA	70	8	7	11
Rasmussen and Olesen[19]	80; 59 MO, 21 MA	53 MO / 33 MA	43 MO / 62 MA	4 MO / 5 MA	NR
Granella et al[20]	943	67 (17 complete remission)	29	4	1
Cupini et al[21]	151: 116 MO, 35 MA	43 MO / 40 MA	53 MO / 53 MA	4 MO / 7 MA	0 MO / 6 MA
Russell et al[22]	110: 87 MO, 33 MA	69 MO / 61 MA	28 MO / 33 MA	3 MO / 6 MA	NR
MacGregor et al[23]	30	53	27	0	1 case MO
Bille[24]	28	85	NR	NR	NR
Maggioni et al[7]	93: 81 MO, 12 MA	86 MO (32 complete remission) / 83 MA (25 complete remission)	10 MO / 17 MA	4 MO / 0 MA	1 case MO / 0 MA
Mattsson et al[25]	125; 102 MO, 23 MA	81 MO / 78 MA	18 MO / 4 MA	1 MO / 17 MA	NR
Granella et al[26]	138: 99 MO; 39 MA	77 MO / 44 MA / OR 0.2 (95% CI 0.1–0.5)	22 MO / 49 MA / OR 3.3 (95% CI 1.4 to 7.90)	1 MO / 8 MA / OR 8.2 (95% CI 0.6–432.9)	NR
Kelman[27]	309	38 (20 complete remission)	28	34	NA

Abbreviations: CI, confidence interval; M, migraine; MA, migraine with aura; MM, menstrual migraine; MO, migraine without aura; NA, not applicable; NR, not reported; NS, not significant; OR, odds ratio; TH, tension headache.

Table 2
Prospective studies of the effect of pregnancy on migraine

Study	No. of Pregnant Migraineurs	Outcome			
		Improved (%)	No Change (%)	Increased (%)	New Onset (%)
Chen and Leviton[28]	484	79 (17 complete remission)	21	NR	NA
Scharff et al[29]	30: 11 migraine; 8 TTH; 11 migraine + TTH	57	37	7	37
Marcus et al[30]	49: 16 migraine; 16 TTH; 15 migraine + TTH	41	NR	NR	28
Sances et al[31]	49: 47 MO; 2 MA	87 MO (79 complete remission) 0 MA	23 MO 100 MA	0 MO 0 MA	NA
Melhado et al[32]	993 women with headaches (848 migraine)	63	27	9	NA
Ertresvag et al[8]	410	66 (50 had nonmigraine headache, 8 complete remission)	20	14	1.9

Abbreviations: MA, migraine with aura; MO, migraine without aura; NA, not applicable; NR, not reported; TTH, tension headache.

Table 3
Outcome of migraine during pregnancy by trimester

Study	Sample Size	First Trimester	Second Trimester	Third Trimester
			Improvement (%)	
Maggioni et al[7]	93: 81 MO, 12 MA	78 MO 67 MA	74 MO 83 MA	83 MO 75 MA
Marcus et al[30]	49: 16 migraine; 16 TTH; 15 migraine + TTH	8	30 improvement between second & third trimesters	
Sances et al[31]	49: 47 MO; 2 MA	47 MO (11 complete remission) 0 MA	83 MO (53 complete remission) 0 MA	87 MO (79 complete remission) 0 MA
Melhado et al[32]	993 women with headaches (848 migraine)	51	60	63

Abbreviations: MA, migraine with aura; MO, migraine without aura; TTH, tension-type headache.

A prospective study of 47 women with migraine without aura prepregnancy noted that attack severity decreased ($P = .001$) in the 20% of women who continued to have migraine throughout pregnancy, although duration of attacks was unchanged.[31] By contrast, in a prospective study of 208 women with migraine attacks during pregnancy, attacks were reported to be of a shorter duration compared with prepregnancy ($P<.001$).[33]

The number of pregnancies has an inverse effect on the benefit of pregnancy on migraine. In the Norwegian Head-HUNT study, adjusting for age and educational level,

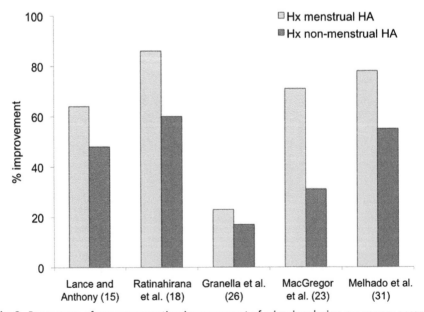

Fig. 2. Percentage of women reporting improvement of migraine during pregnancy according to type of migraine.

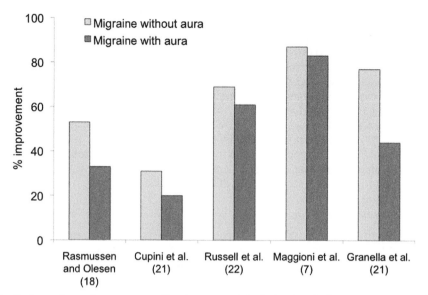

Fig. 3. Percentage of women reporting improvement of migraine during pregnancy according to prepregnant history of menstrual headache.

the 1-year prevalence of migraine in 9281 women 40 years or younger was lower in pregnant than in nonpregnant women.[9] The association was significant for women pregnant with their first child (OR 0.5, 95% CI 0.3–0.9), but not for multiparous women (OR 0.8, 95% CI 0.6–1.1). Of 20,287 nonpregnant women who were 70 years or younger, women without children had significantly fewer migraines than women with children (OR 1.3, 95% CI 1.2–1.5).

New-onset transient neurologic symptoms may occur during pregnancy and are more likely to affect women with preexisting migraine than women with nonmigraine headaches or no headache.[8,21,34] A case-control study assessed 41 pregnant women with transient focal neurologic deficits and 41 pregnant controls.[35] Thirty-four cases were diagnosed with migraine aura and 2 cases with stroke. For many of the cases diagnosed with migraine, it was their first-ever attack.

Another case-control study enrolled 14 pregnant women with acute transient focal neurologic symptoms who had no history of migraine, recurrent thromboembolism, or cerebrovascular disease, and compared them with 28 symptom-free control patients.[36] Mean gestational age at symptom onset was 28 (range 17–44) weeks. Presenting symptoms included dysphasia (n = 6), hemisensory (n = 5), and hemimotor (n = 7) symptoms. Four patients experienced scintillating scotoma and in 9 patients, symptoms were followed by a first-ever, throbbing, migraine-like headache. Only one patient had evidence of frank infarction on magnetic resonance imaging (MRI); 2 patients had single, small, hyperintense bright foci on fluid-attenuated inversion-recovery imaging without accompanying lesions on diffusion-weighted imaging, and 11 patients had normal MRI and magnetic resonance venography results. Echocardiography, carotid duplex ultrasonography, and hypercoagulability results were negative in all patients. None of the patients had ischemic events. Four (29%) developed migraines with aura headaches during follow-up.

Diagnosis of migraine may be difficult, as aura features tend to be complex.[35] New-onset hemiplegic migraine, presenting with unilateral weakness associated with long-duration aura, has also been reported during pregnancy.[37]

Postpartum Headaches

Headache is common in the week following delivery, affecting around 30% to 40% of women.[29,31,33,38–40] In a prospective cohort study of 985 deliveries, 381 (39%) women reported postpartum headaches or neck/shoulder pain.[40] The median time to onset of headache was 2 days (0, 6; first and third quartiles) and duration was 4 hours (2, 24; first and third quartiles). Primary headaches accounted for more than 70% of all headaches (tension-type headache 38.3%, migrainous 26.8%, migraine without aura 6.3%, migraine with aura 1%), musculoskeletal and cervicogenic headache accounted for 14.7%, postdural puncture headache accounted for 4.7%, and 8.1% were undetermined. The most significant risk factors for the development of postpartum headache were inadvertent dural puncture, previous headache history, multiparity, shorter pushing in second stage of labor, and increased maternal age.

Headaches During Lactation

Breastfeeding should be encouraged, as it generally sustains the benefits of pregnancy on migraine. A longitudinal prospective study of headache during pregnancy and postpartum found that the headache index during the first 3 postpartum months was similar for patients who breastfed to that obtained during the second trimester of pregnancy.[30] A study of 49 women with migraine reported that migraine recurred within the first postpartum month in 100% of women who bottle-fed and in only 43.2% of those who breastfed ($P = .0003$).[31] The protective effect of breastfeeding probably relates to stable low levels of estrogen because lactation inhibits ovulation, with the mean time to ovulation after delivery being 189 days in breastfeeding women and 45 days in non-breastfeeding women.[41]

EFFECT OF PRIMARY HEADACHES ON PREGNANCY AND LACTATION
Outcome of Pregnancy

The majority of studies confirms that migraine with or without aura is not associated with significant adverse effects on the outcome of pregnancy. In a retrospective study of 450 migraineurs who had had 1142 pregnancies and 136 controls who had had 342 pregnancies, the incidence of miscarriage or stillbirth was similar, both overall (17% migraineurs vs 18% controls) and during the first trimester (13% migraineurs vs 13% controls).[42] The incidence of birth defects was also similar for both groups (3.35% migraineurs vs 3.96% controls).

A study in Hungary evaluated 22,843 newborns or fetuses with congenital abnormalities, 38,151 control newborn infants without any abnormalities, and 834 controls with Down syndrome.[43] Migraine during pregnancy affected 565 (2.5%) mothers of the group with congenital abnormalities versus 713 (1.9%) mothers in the normal group (crude prevalence odds ratio [POR] 1.3, 95% CI 1.2–1.5) and 24 (2.9%) pregnant women in the Down syndrome control group (crude POR 0.9, 95% CI 0.6–1.3). Of all the parameters studied, the only positive finding was that limb deficiencies were associated with a higher rate of maternal migraines during the first trimester of pregnancy, for both the congenital abnormalities group versus the matched normal group (adjusted POR 2.5, 95% CI 1.1–5.8) and the congenital abnormalities group versus Down syndrome controls (adjusted POR 1.7, 95% CI 1.3–3.0). Although this study has the benefit of large numbers, allowing rare events to be identified, these data are not confirmatory and the effect of other independent variables, drug and nondrug treatments taken, and misdiagnosis of conditions mimicking migraine cannot be ruled out.

There is limited evidence that migraine is associated with an increased risk of low birth weight. In a case-control study in Taiwan of 4911 women with migraine who gave birth between 2001 and 2003, multivariate logistic regression analyses showed that after adjusting for potential confounders, babies born to women with migraine were at increased risk of low birth weight (OR 1.16, 95% CI 1.03–1.31, P = .014) and preterm birth (OR 1.24, 95% CI 1.13–1.39, P<.001) compared with 24,555 matched controls.[44] An analysis of the Pharmaco-Epidemiological Prescription Database of North Jutland County between 1991 and 1996 identified 34 women who took sumatriptan during pregnancy, and using logistic regression models their pregnancy outcome was compared with 89 pregnant migraine controls, defined as migraine patients who did not redeem prescriptions for migraine treatment during pregnancy, and 15,955 healthy pregnant women.[45] The risk of a low-birth-weight infant was increased (OR 3.0, 95% CI 1.3–7.0) for all migraine patients who delivered at term (n = 115) compared with the outcome of healthy pregnancies. The risk of preterm delivery was raised only in women who took sumatriptan: OR 6.3 (95% CI 1.2–32.0) compared with migraine controls and OR 3.3 (95% CI 1.3–8.5) compared with healthy women.

By contrast, an analysis of a population-based data set of 713 women who had severe migraine during pregnancy, mean gestational age and birth weight, as well as the proportion of low-birth-weight and preterm births, were similar in newborn infants born to mothers with or without migraine.[46]

If low birth weight is associated with migraine, it may be the consequence of comorbid conditions rather than migraine itself. In a cohort study of 3432 pregnant women, women with comorbid migraine and mood disorder were almost twice as likely to deliver preterm compared with the reference group with no migraine or mood disorder (adjusted relative risk [RR] 1.87, 95% CI 1.05–3.34).[4] There was no increased risk of preterm delivery with migraine only (adjusted RR 0.86, 95% CI 0.61–1.21) or with mood disorder only (adjusted RR 1.56, 95% CI 0.98–2.47).

Risk of Vascular Disorders

An increasing body of evidence supports an association between migraine, pregnancy-induced hypertension, and preeclampsia (**Table 4**).[47] A case-control study of 244 women with preeclampsia and 470 normotensive controls found that a history of migraine was associated with a 1.8-fold increased risk of preeclampsia (95% CI 1.1–2.7). Women who were 30 years or older when diagnosed with migraine had the highest risk (OR 2.8, 95% CI 0.8–9.0).[48] Obesity was an additional risk factor, as overweight migraineurs had a 12-fold increased risk of preeclampsia (95% CI 5.9–25.7) compared with lean women without migraine.

A cohort study of 3432 pregnant women assessed risk of hypertensive disorder of pregnancy in women with migraine and/or mood disorder compared with controls without either condition.[4] Women with mood disorder alone had elevated risks of preeclampsia compared with controls (adjusted RR 3.57, 95% CI 1.83–6.99) as did women with migraine and mood disorders (adjusted RR 3.49, 95% CI 1.07–11.36). Migraine alone was not associated with increased risk of preeclampsia (adjusted RR 1.08, 95% CI 0.55–2.15) but was associated with increased risk of pregnancy-induced hypertension (adjusted RR 1.42, 95% CI 1.00–2.01). There was no increased risk of pregnancy-induced hypertension in women with mood disorder alone (adjusted RR 0.91, 95% CI 0.44–1.86) or comorbid migraine and mood disorder (adjusted RR 1.86, 95% CI 0.82–4.24) compared with controls.

Migraine has also been identified as a risk factor for pregnancy-related stroke. Pregnancy and 6 weeks postpartum are prothrombotic states for all women, with an incidence of pregnancy-related stroke between 11 and 26 per 100,000 deliveries and

Table 4
Risk of pregnancy-induced hypertension and preeclampsia

Study	Type	Sample Size	Pregnancy-Induced Hypertension	Preeclampsia
Wainscott et al[42]	Case-control	450 migraineurs, 136 controls		Risk of toxemia in cases vs controls: 18% vs 18%
Moore and Redman[76]	Case-control	24 cases of preeclampsia, 48 controls		Risk of headache in cases vs controls: 34% vs 6% (P<.01)
Marcoux et al[77]	Case-control	426 cases (172 preeclampsia; 254 pregnancy-induced hypertension). 505 controls	OR 1.70 (95% CI 1.02–2.85)	OR 2.44 (95% CI 1.42–4.20)
Mattsson et al[25]	Cross-sectional	685 migraineurs	Risk of MO: adjusted OR[a] 1.26 (95% CI 0.78–1.99) Risk of MA: adjusted OR[a] 0.97 (95% CI 0.38–2.13)	
Facchinetti et al[78]	Case-control	75 cases with recent preeclampsia, 75 controls with uneventful pregnancy at term		Risk of headache in cases vs controls: OR 4.95 (95% CI 2.47–9.92) 44/47 cases with headache had migraine; 13/19 controls with headache had migraine
Scher et al[79]	Case-control	482 migraineurs, 2517 controls	Risk of migraine: adjusted OR[b] 1.63 (95% CI 1.2–2.1) (P<.05) Risk of MO: adjusted OR[b] 1.63 (95% CI 1.0–2.6) Risk of MA: adjusted OR[b] 1.64 (95% CI 1.2–2.3)	

Study	Design	Population	Adjusted results	Main findings
Adeney et al[48]	Case-control	244 cases with preeclampsia vs 470 normotensive controls		Risk of migraine in cases vs controls: OR 1.8 (95% CI 1.1–2.7)
Banhidy et al[43]	Case-control	38151 newborn infants of which 713 mothers had severe migraine during pregnancy		Risk of migraine in cases vs controls: POR 1.4 (95% CI 1.1–1.8)
Facchinetti et al[80]	Prospective cohort study	270 women with migraine, 432 controls	Adjusted OR[c] 2.85 (95% CI 1.40–5.81)	
Sanchez et al[81]	Case-control	339 cases with preeclampsia vs 337 normotensive controls		Risk of preeclampsia in women with migraine during pregnancy vs controls: OR 4.0 (95% CI 1.9–8.2)
Chen et al[44]	Case-control	4911 women with migraine, 24555 controls		Risk of preeclampsia in women with migraine during pregnancy vs controls: OR 1.34 (95% CI 1.02–1.77)

Abbreviations: CI, confidence interval; OR, odds ratio; POR, prevalence odds ratio.
[a] Adjusted for age.
[b] Adjusted for age, socioecomonic status, smoking, and alcohol intake.
[c] Adjusted for age, family history of hypertension, and smoking.

a mortality of 10% to 13%.[49] Analysis of data from the Nationwide Inpatient Sample from the Healthcare Cost and Utilization Project of the Agency for Healthcare Research and Quality identified 2850 pregnancy-related discharges for the years 2000 to 2001.[50] The stroke rate was 34.2 per 100,000 deliveries and the mortality rate was 1.4 per 100,000 deliveries. Migraine was associated with an increased risk of preeclampsia/pregnancy-induced hypertension (OR 4.4, 95% CI 3.6–5.4) and stroke (OR 16.9, 95% CI 9.7–29.5).

Analysis of the same database for the years 2000 to 2003 identified 33,956 women with migraine. Women with migraine during pregnancy had an increased risk of stroke (OR 15.05, 95% CI 8.26–27.4), myocardial infarction/heart disease (OR 2.11, 95% CI 1.76–2.54), pulmonary embolus/venous thromboembolism (OR 3.23, 95% CI 2.06–7.07), hypertension (OR 8.61, 95% CI 6.43–11.54), preeclampsia/pregnancy-induced hypertension (2.29, 2.13–2.46), smoking (OR 2.85, 95% 2.53–3.21), and diabetes (OR 1.96, 95% 1.64–2.35). Although these findings suggest a strong association between migraine during pregnancy and increased risk of vascular disease, further research is necessary to identify differences in risk between migraine with aura and migraine without aura, and to ascertain if migraine is an independent risk factor for stroke, or if risk factors for arterial disease are associated with increased risk of migraine.

Secondary Headaches

Headache during pregnancy results from the same reasons as headache occurring in nonpregnant women. Secondary causes of headache more likely to occur as a consequence of pregnancy include eclampsia, stroke, postdural puncture headache, cerebral angiopathy, pituitary apoplexy, and cerebral venous thrombosis. A careful history and examination usually leads to the diagnosis of the underlying cause. Identifying "red flags" is important, as these indicate the need for urgent assessment (**Fig. 4**).[37,51]

In women presenting with aura for the first time during pregnancy, thrombocytopenia, cerebral venous sinus thrombosis, or imminent eclampsia should be excluded. Gradually developing symptoms, or different symptoms occurring in succession as described in the International Classification of Headache Disorders, are distinguishing features of migraine aura.[35]

INVESTIGATIONS FOR HEADACHE IN PREGNANCY AND LACTATION

Routine investigations should be deferred until after delivery. The majority of headaches can be diagnosed from the history and examination without the need for investigations, which are indicated only to exclude suspected secondary headache resulting from underlying abnormality. Should investigations be required, they are the same as for nonpregnant women. Most diagnostic radiologic procedures are associated with little, if any, significant fetal risks. The American College of Obstetricians and Gynecologists regard x-ray exposure from a single diagnostic procedure as harmful although MRI, which is considered safe in pregnancy, is preferred.[52] Contrast imaging can be undertaken if indicated. Although no adverse fetal effects follow the use of gadolinium, iodinated contrast media has the potential to depress thyroid function. If used, neonatal thyroid function should be checked during the first week.[53] Breastfeeding can continue without restriction, as only minimal iodinated or gadolinium-based contrast medium is excreted in milk and only minute amounts are absorbed by the baby.[53]

MANAGEMENT OF HEADACHE DURING PREGNANCY AND LACTATION

The options for management are drugs to treat acute symptoms, drugs to prevent attacks, and nonpharmacologic interventions to prevent attacks. These agents can

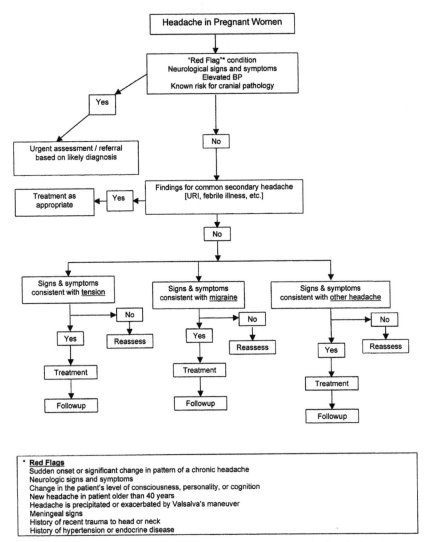

Fig. 4. Recognizing red flags is an important factor in diagnosing headaches in pregnant women. BP, blood pressure; URI, upper respiratory infection. (*From* Von Wald T, Walling AD. Headache during pregnancy. Obstet Gynecol Surv 2002;57:179–85; and Reproduced with permission from Lippincott Williams & Wilkins, Inc.)

be used alone or in combination, depending on headache frequency and individual preferences.

Nonpharmacologic

Nonpharmacologic treatment has the obvious benefit of minimal risk to mother and fetus. It should be considered as the initial step in the management of tension-type headache or migraine but is ineffective for cluster headache, which can only be controlled with medication.

As in the nonpregnant state, information, reassurance, and coping with trigger factors help reduce the frequency of headache.[54] The most frequently reported triggers are stress (mental or physical), irregular or inappropriate meals, high intake or withdrawal of coffee and other caffeine-containing drinks, dehydration, sleep disorders, too much or too little sleep, and reduced or excessive physical exercise.[6,55] These triggers can be controlled with adequate sleep, regular nourishment and hydration, and moderate physical exercise. Alcohol and smoking are potentially harmful to the fetus and should be avoided during pregnancy.

A meta-analysis of 53 studies has confirmed the efficacy of biofeedback, particularly electromyography (EMG) biofeedback, and muscle-relaxation training for tension-type headache.[56] In a study assessing the effects a combination of relaxation, biofeedback, and physical therapy in pregnant women with migraine, 79% reported improvement.[57] The benefits of these interventions may be maintained beyond pregnancy.[58]

There is evidence for efficacy of acupuncture for migraine and tension-type headache, which also treats nausea and vomiting in pregnancy.[59–61]

A randomized trial of 300 mg coenzyme Q10 daily showed efficacy for migraine prophylaxis and, although there are no data for this indication from trials undertaken in pregnancy, a randomized trial of 200 mg daily taken by women at risk of preeclampsia from 20 weeks of pregnancy to delivery was associated with a significant reduced risk of preeclampsia.[62,63] Similarly, magnesium supplements, which can be used for migraine prophylaxis, can halve the risk of eclampsia with no evidence of adverse effects on pregnancy.[64,65]

Pharmacologic

Most drugs and other teratogens exert their greatest effects on the fetus in the first trimester, often before pregnancy is confirmed. Drug use during pregnancy is common, and many women continue to use their usual headache medication, including triptans, throughout pregnancy.[66] To avoid the potential for drug-related effects on pregnancy, it is important to minimize drug exposure in any woman who is planning pregnancy or who is at high risk of unplanned pregnancy. If possible, prophylactic medication should be discontinued and strategies for the management of acute attacks discussed. As few drugs as possible should be used, which have the least potential to cause damage, at the lowest effective dose. Although many of the drugs taken by unsuspecting pregnant women rarely cause harm, there is a difference between reassuring the pregnant woman that what she has taken is unlikely to have affected the pregnancy and advising her as to what is safe and effective treatment for future attacks. Most evidence of safety is circumstantial; few drugs have been tested during pregnancy and lactation because of the obvious ethical limitations of undertaking clinical trials. This lack of data means that use of most drugs in pregnancy is unlicensed, so drugs should be considered only if the potential benefits to the woman and fetus outweigh the potential risks. The woman should be given sufficient information about any known risks, and make her own decision about drug use, with clear documentation of the discussion.

Recommendations for pharmacologic treatment of primary headaches during pregnancy and lactation

Tension-type headache Symptomatic treatment using simple analgesics and nonsteroidal anti-inflammatory drugs (NSAIDs) is the mainstay of management of episodic tension-type headache during pregnancy and lactation.[67] Paracetamol is the analgesic of choice during pregnancy. Aspirin and NSAIDs can be taken in the first and second trimesters but should be avoided near term. Although NSAIDs are safe during lactation, aspirin should be avoided. Triptans, muscle relaxants, and opioids are of no benefit and may increase the risk of medication-overuse headache. Prophylactic medications are seldom necessary and are only indicated for chronic tension-type headache or when headaches regularly occur more than 2 to 3 days a week. Amitriptyline is the prophylactic drug of first choice for prophylaxis of tension-type headache during pregnancy and lactation.[67]

Cluster headache Medication is essential for effective management of cluster headache, and both symptomatic and prophylactic treatment is usually necessary to gain effective control. Preferred treatments during pregnancy and lactation are oxygen, subcutaneous or intranasal sumatriptan for acute treatment, and verapamil or prednisone/prednisolone for prophylaxis.[68] There are no safety concerns regarding use of oxygen during pregnancy, even at hyperbaric pressures.[69] Gabapentin is a second-line prophylactic option during pregnancy and lactation. Lithium is an additional option for prophylaxis during lactation, but should not be used during pregnancy.

Migraine Analgesics can be used, as for tension-type headache. Most antiemetics can be continued throughout pregnancy and lactation. Sumatriptan may be indicated for severe attacks during pregnancy that do not respond to first-line drugs, and can be used during lactation without disruption to breastfeeding. If prophylaxis is indicated during pregnancy or lactation, the lowest effective dose of propranolol is the first-line recommendation. Amitriptyline is also an option.

EVIDENCE FOR SAFETY OF DRUGS IN PREGNANCY AND LACTATION

There are several sources in the United States that provide information on safety of drugs during pregnancy and lactation, listed under "Resources." These resources provided the evidence for the recommendations listed here. The US Food and Drugs Administration (FDA) pregnancy labeling has 5 categories: A, B, C, D, and X (**Box 1**). These categories can be misleading, as categories C, D, and X are not only based on risk but consider risk versus benefit, so drugs in each of the 3 categories may pose similar risks. Furthermore, the categories do not always differentiate between human or animal data or consider differences in frequency, severity, and type of fetal toxicities in relation to background risk, nor do they provide information on lactation. The FDA proposes to withdraw these categories in favor of separate sections for pregnancy and lactation. Each section contains a summary statement on risk, followed by clinical considerations and other relevant information. This information is provided by the UK Teratology Information Service, which provides summaries from preclinical and human studies for individual drugs.

DRUGS TAKEN FOR HEADACHES DURING PREGNANCY AND LACTATION

This section reviews drugs used for the acute treatment (**Table 5**) and prophylactic treatment (**Table 6**) of headache.

Acute Treatment of Headache

Analgesics
Acetaminophen Data from large cohort and case-control studies confirm the safety of therapeutic doses ($\leq$4 g/d) of acetaminophen during pregnancy and lactation. It is the analgesic of choice for the short-term relief of mild to moderate pain and pyrexia.

Box 1
FDA pregnancy categories

Category A

Adequate and well-controlled studies have failed to demonstrate a risk to the fetus in the first trimester of pregnancy (and there is no evidence of risk in later trimesters).

Category B

Animal reproduction studies have failed to demonstrate a risk to the fetus and there are no adequate and well-controlled studies in pregnant women.

Category C

Animal reproduction studies have shown an adverse effect on the fetus and there are no adequate and well-controlled studies in humans, but potential benefits may warrant use of the drug in pregnant women despite potential risks.

Category D

There is positive evidence of human fetal risk based on adverse reaction data from investigational or marketing experience or studies in humans, but potential benefits may warrant use of the drug in pregnant women despite potential risks.

Category X

Studies in animals or humans have demonstrated fetal abnormalities and/or there is positive evidence of human fetal risk based on adverse reaction data from investigational or marketing experience, and the risks involved in use of the drug in pregnant women clearly outweigh potential benefits.

Aspirin Clinical and epidemiologic data from large numbers of women who have taken analgesic doses of aspirin during pregnancy provide evidence of its safety in the first and second trimesters. Although numerous malformations have been reported following maternal use of aspirin during pregnancy, with the exception of a possible risk of gastroschisis, no specific pattern of malformations has been observed and a causative role for aspirin has not been proved. Aspirin should be used with caution near term, as its effect on platelet function increases the risk of prolonged labor, postpartum hemorrhage, and neonatal bleeding. In common with NSAIDs, aspirin may be associated with premature closure of the fetal ductus arteriosus. Because aspirin is excreted in breast milk, breastfeeding mothers should avoid regular use because of the theoretical risk of Reye syndrome and impaired platelet function in susceptible infants, although occasional use by the mother is unlikely to cause adverse effects.

Nonsteroidal anti-inflammatory drugs There are insufficient data to support the use of NSAIDs other than ibuprofen, which is the preferred NSAID during pregnancy and can be given in doses not exceeding 600 mg daily. The available data do not indicate that exposure to ibuprofen before 30 weeks of pregnancy is associated with an increased risk of malformations or spontaneous miscarriage. Chronic exposure or exposure to high doses after 30 weeks is associated with an increased risk of premature closure of the ductus arteriosus and oligohydramnios, which is related to the inhibitory effect of ibuprofen on prostaglandin activity. In circumstances whereby the clinical condition requires treatment with NSAIDs during the third trimester, the fetus should be monitored regularly to detect any potential adverse effects. During lactation, the concentration of NSAIDs in breast milk is very low and is unlikely to affect the infant.

Table 5
Drugs used for acute treatment of headache

	FDA Category	Recommendation in Pregnancy	Recommendation in Lactation	Notes
Analgesics				
Acetaminophen	B	✓	✓	First-line Amounts in breast milk are much less than doses usually given to infants
Aspirin	C (first & second trimesters) D (third trimester)	✓	✗	Second-line Avoid from 30 weeks
Diclofenac	B (first & second trimesters) D (third trimester)	✓	✓	Second-line Short half-life Avoid from 30 weeks
Ibuprofen	B (first & second trimesters) D (third trimester)	✓	✓	Second-line NSAID of choice Short half-life Avoid from 30 weeks Amounts in breast milk are much less than doses usually given to infants
Indomethacin	B (first & second trimesters) D (third trimester)	(✓)	(✓)	Avoid from 30 weeks Used therapeutically in infants but drugs with more data of use in lactation preferred
Mefenamic acid	C (first & second trimesters) D (third trimester)	(✓)	✗	Avoid from 30 weeks Drugs with more data of use in lactation preferred
Naproxen	B (first & second trimesters) D (third trimester)	(✓)	(✓)	Avoid from 30 weeks Drugs with short half-life preferred

(continued on next page)

Table 5
(continued)

	FDA Category	Recommendation in Pregnancy	Recommendation in Lactation	Notes
Opiates				
Codeine	C	(✓)	(✓)	Opiates not recommended for migraine Monitor baby for withdrawal symptoms postpartum May cause infant sedation Nonnarcotic analgesic preferred
Morphine	C	(✓)	(✓)	Opiates not recommended for migraine Infant may have measurable blood concentration May cause infant sedation Nonnarcotic analgesic preferred
Pethidine/ meperidine	B	(✓)	(✓)	Opiates not recommended for migraine Category D if prolonged use/high doses at term Monitor baby for withdrawal symptoms postpartum
Tramadol	C	(✓)	(✓)	
Barbiturates				
Butalbital	C	✗	✗	Category D if used in high doses at term or for prolonged periods
Phenobarbital	D	✗	✗	Sedation, infantile spasms after weaning from milk containing phenobarbital
Antiemetics				
Cyclizine	B	✓	✓	First-line

Drug	FDA			Comment
Domperidone	C	(✓)	✓	Fewer data in pregnancy than for other antiemetics
Metoclopramide	B	✓	✓	
Prochlorperazine	C	✓	✓	
Promethazine	C	✓	✓	First-line
Triptans				
Almotriptan	C	ID	ID	
Eletriptan	C	ID	(✓)	
Frovatriptan	C	ID	ID	Long half-life; drugs with short half-life preferred
Naratriptan	C	ID	ID	
Sumatriptan	C	✓	✓	Third-line
				Consider for severe unresponsive attacks
Rizatriptan	C	ID	ID	
Zolmitriptan	C	ID	ID	
Ergots				
Ergotamine	X	✗	✗	Contraindicated
Dihydroergotamine	X	✗	✗	Contraindicated

Abbreviations: ✓, minimal risk; (✓), benefits likely to outweigh risks; ✗, not recommended; FDA, US Food and Drug Administration; ID, insufficient data; NSAID, nonsteroidal anti-inflammatory drug.

Table 6
Drugs used for prophylactic treatment of headache

	FDA Category	Recommendation in Pregnancy	Recommendation in Lactation	Notes
Antiplatelet drugs				
Aspirin	C	✓	✓	Doses ≤150 mg daily
Tricyclics				
Amitriptyline	C	✓	✓	Monitor baby for withdrawal symptoms Low levels in breast milk
Nortriptyline	Not classified	✓	✓	Monitor baby for withdrawal symptoms Low levels in breast milk
SSRI/SNRIs				
Citalopram	C	(✓)	✗	Amitriptyline or nortriptyline preferred Infant exposure lower with escitalopram
Escitalopram	C	(✓)	(✓)	Amitriptyline or nortriptyline preferred Infant exposure lower than with citalopram
Fluoxetine	C	(✓)	✗	Amitriptyline or nortriptyline preferred Higher levels in breast milk than other SSRIs and long-acting metabolite Other SSRIs preferred unless patient established on treatment Monitor infant
Paroxetine	D	✗	(✓)	Amitriptyline or nortriptyline preferred First-trimester use associated with increased risk of cardiovascular malformations Low levels in breast milk
Sertraline	C	(✓)	(✓)	Amitriptyline or nortriptyline preferred Low levels in breast milk No adverse reactions attributed
Venlafaxine	C	(✓)	(✓)	Amitriptyline or nortriptyline preferred Excreted into breast milk

Drug	Category			Comments
β-Blockers				
Atenolol	D	x	x	Propranolol or metoprolol preferred
Metoprolol	C	(✓)	(✓)	Low levels in breast milk
Nadolol	C	(✓)	x	Other β-adrenergic blocking drugs preferred
Propranolol	C	✓	✓	β-Blocker of choice Low levels in breast milk No adverse reactions attributed
Timolol	C	(✓)	x	Propranolol or metoprolol preferred Variable excretion into breast milk Limited data
Calcium-channel blockers				
Flunarizine	Not classified	ID	ID	
Verapamil	C	✓	✓	No data on high doses in pregnancy Doses up to 360 mg daily produce low serum levels in infant but no adverse reactions attributed
Nifedipine	C	x	✓	
Angiotensin II antagonists				
Candesartan	C (first trimester) D (second/third trimesters)	x	ID	Contraindicated Evidence of fetal toxicity
Angiotensin-converting enzyme inhibitors				
Lisinopril	C (first trimester) D (second/third trimesters)	x	ID	Teratogenic
Antiepileptics				
Gabapentin	C	ID	(✓)	Doses up to 2.1 g daily produce relatively low levels in infant serum Monitor infant for side effects
Topiramate	D	x	(✓)	Doses up to 200 mg daily produce relatively low levels in infant serum Monitor infant for side effects

(continued on next page)

Table 6
(continued)

	FDA Category	Recommendation in Pregnancy	Recommendation in Lactation	Notes
Valproic acid	D	x	(✓)	Contraindicated in pregnancy as teratogenic. Low levels in infant serum. Theoretical risk of infant hepatotoxicity. Monitor for jaundice
Other drugs				
Botulinum toxin	C	ID	ID	
Lithium	D	x	x	Teratogenic
Methysergide	X	x	x	No longer available in USA

Abbreviations: ✓, minimal risk; (✓), benefits likely to outweigh risks; x, not recommended; FDA, US Food and Drug Administration; ID, insufficient data; SNRI, serotonin-norepinephrine reuptake inhibitor; SSRI, selective serotonin reuptake inhibitor.

Opiates

Opiates have been widely used during pregnancy for many years without apparent ill consequence. Although they are used to treat moderate to severe pain, they are inappropriate for migraine because they aggravate nausea and reduce gastric motility. Chronic use of opiates in later pregnancy has been associated with neonatal withdrawal symptoms.

Adverse effects during lactation are unlikely. However, some women metabolize opiates differently, which can cause higher levels of opiates to pass into their breast milk, resulting in drowsiness and sedation.

Barbiturates

There are only limited human data for butalbital during pregnancy, and no human data from treatment during lactation. Phenobarbital has been associated with teratogenicity, and can cause neonatal withdrawal and hemorrhagic disease of the newborn. It is excreted into breast milk and accumulates in infants' blood, causing sedation and withdrawal symptoms.

Antiemetics

First-line antiemetics of choice in pregnancy and lactation are cyclizine and promethazine. Prochlorperazine and metoclopramide can also be used, but with an increased risk of maternal dystonic reactions. Metoclopramide has the advantage of reversing gastric stasis in migraine. During lactation, doses of 10 to 15 mg 3 times daily can increase milk production by up to 100%. Higher doses should not be used. The amount of metoclopramide transferred into breast milk is small. There are only limited data for domperidone in pregnancy, but it can be used during lactation. Like metoclopramide, domperidone is a dopamine agonist that stimulates prolactin. Mean milk volume can increase by more than 40% over 7 days. Domperidone does not cross the blood-brain barrier, so it is not associated with extrapyramidal side effects. Transfer of domperidone into breast milk is minimal.

Triptans

Sumatriptan There is no evidence of a large increased risk of congenital malformations or other adverse pregnancy outcomes from exposure to sumatriptan at any stage in pregnancy. Therefore, if clinically appropriate, sumatriptan may be considered for the acute treatment of migraine during pregnancy (see Case Study). However, the possibility of a small increase in risk of a specific birth defect cannot be excluded. Data from the Sumatriptan/Naratriptan/Treximet Pregnancy Registry (1 January, 1996 to 31 October, 2010) are reassuring, and confirm that inadvertent exposure to sumatriptan during pregnancy has not been associated with adverse outcomes. The observed proportion with birth defects following earliest exposure in the first trimester was 20 of 462 (ie, 4.3%; 95% CI 2.7%–6.7%). The observed proportion with birth defects found outcomes with any trimester of exposure was 24 of 554 (4.3%; 95% CI 2.9%–6.5%). This figure compares favorably with the 3% to 5% risk of birth defects in the general population.

The low level of excretion of sumatriptan in breast milk suggests that continued breastfeeding following its use does not pose a significant risk to the infant. Five women who had been breastfeeding for 11 to 28 weeks received a single dose of sumatriptan, 6 mg by subcutaneous injection. The peak milk level averaged 87.2 µg/L (range 62–113 µg/L), which occurred 2.5 hours (range 1.7–3.5 hours) after the dose. The mean half-life in milk was 2.2 hours (range 1.2–3.1 hours). The investigators calculated that an exclusively breastfed infant would receive 14.4 µg sumatriptan in breast milk with this dose, which is 3.5% of the weight-adjusted dosage.[70] The American Academy of Pediatrics considered that sumatriptan can be used without restriction of breastfeeding.[71] This recommendation is contrary to the prescribing information, which cautions that "infant exposure can be minimized by avoiding breastfeeding for 12 hours after treatment."

Naratriptan Data from the Sumatriptan/Naratriptan/Treximet Pregnancy Registry (1 January, 1996 to 31 October, 2010) includes 52 pregnancies with first-trimester exposure to naratriptan. One live infant with a birth defect was reported, who had also had first-trimester exposure to sumatriptan. An additional 5 pregnancies following earliest exposure during the second trimester resulted in 5 live births with no defects reported. The prescribing data states only that "caution should be exercised when considering administration of naratriptan to breastfeeding women."

Rizatriptan Data from the 94 women enrolled in the rizatriptan Pregnancy Registry (June 1998 to 31 July, 2009) and reports from other sources do not suggest that treatment during pregnancy predisposes patients to spontaneous miscarriages or congenital anomalies above the normal rate. However, the number of reports is small. It is not known whether rizatriptan is excreted in human milk. The prescribing information advises caution if rizatriptan is administered to women who are breastfeeding.

Other triptans There are insufficient data on other triptans during pregnancy. In one study of 8 women given a single 80-mg oral dose of eletriptan, the mean total amount of eletriptan in breast milk over 24 hours was only 0.02% of the administered dose. It is not known whether almotriptan, frovatriptan, or zolmitriptan are excreted in human milk. The prescribing information advises caution if these drugs are administered to breastfeeding women.

Ergotamine and dihydroergotamine
Inadvertent use of ergotamine during pregnancy has not been associated with any teratogenic effects.[42] However, ergot alkaloids affect uterine hypertonicity and cause vascular disruption, increasing the risk of miscarriage. These agents should not be used during breastfeeding because of reported nausea, vomiting, diarrhea, and weakness in the breastfeeding infant, and suppression of prolactin secretion and lactation in the mother.

Prophylactic Treatment of Headache

Aspirin
One small trial reviewed 28 pregnant women with frequent or severe migraine attacks taking low-dose aspirin (75 mg) for migraine prophylaxis. There was no placebo control but 22 women reported subjective improvement.[72] The investigators base their rationale for using aspirin to prevent migraine on its effect to counteract platelet activation that occurs in pregnancy. Low-dose aspirin has been extensively studied in preeclampsia during pregnancy, with no increase in bleeding complications and negligible effects on the ductus arteriosus observed.

β-Blockers
Use of the β-blocking drugs during pregnancy has not been associated with an increased risk of structural fetal malformations. Some recent studies have suggested a possible increased risk of congenital heart defects, intrauterine growth retardation, and low birth weight associated with β-adrenoceptor blocking drugs, particularly atenolol. However, it is unclear whether these result from the underlying maternal condition or the use of medication. Treatment near term may result in neonatal bradycardia, hypotension, and hypoglycemia. Respiratory distress and apnea have been reported following in utero exposure to β-adrenoceptor blocking agents. The data on the safety of discontinuing treatment 24 to 48 hours before delivery are conflicting. When reported, neonatal symptoms are usually mild and resolve within 48 hours.

Most β-blockers are not significantly excreted into breast milk and can be used during breastfeeding. However, the infant should be monitored in case of bradycardia and hypoglycemia. Propranolol or metoprolol are preferred to atenolol or nadolol, which are associated with relatively extensive excretion into breast milk and extensive renal excretion.

Tricyclic antidepressants

Low-dose amitriptyline or nortriptyline (10–25 mg daily) is also an option. While there are conflicting data regarding limb deformities associated with use of high doses of amitriptyline during pregnancy, there are no reports associated with low doses between 10 and 50 mg daily used for pain management. Tachycardia, irritability, muscle spasms, and convulsion have been reported in neonates of women taking antidepressive doses. The neonate should be monitored for adverse effects such as drowsiness, jitteriness, hyperexcitability, and suckling problems. Where clinically possible, it is recommended that the dose is tapered 3 to 4 weeks before delivery.

Amitriptyline and nortriptyline are barely detectable in breast milk, and low maternal doses are unlikely to affect the infant adversely.

Selective serotonin/noradrenaline reuptake inhibitors

Selective serotonin reuptake inhibitors (SSRIs) used to treat headache include citalopram, escitalopram, fluoxetine, paroxetine, and sertraline. Venlafaxine is a selective serotonin and noradrenaline reuptake inhibitor (SNRI).

Data on the risk of congenital malformations following SSRI/SNRI use in early pregnancy are conflicting. Whereas several studies have demonstrated no statistically significant increase in risk, one large study has suggested an increased risk of cardiovascular malformations. However, if SSRI exposure in pregnancy does cause cardiovascular malformations, the absolute risk appears to be small.

Use of any SSRI in late pregnancy may result in a mild transient neonatal withdrawal syndrome of the central nervous system, motor, respiratory, and gastrointestinal signs. More serious is the potential complication of persistent pulmonary hypertension of the newborn, although the estimated absolute risk is less than 0.5%. This complication has been associated with exposure to SSRIs as a class beyond 20 weeks of gestation.

The rate of venlafaxine/desvenlafaxine excretion into human breast milk is relatively higher than that observed for other antidepressants, largely attributable to higher excretion of the metabolite desvenlafaxine.

Calcium-channel blockers

There are no human data regarding teratogenicity or excretion into breast milk for flunarizine.

Data for verapamil are limited. No association with congenital anomalies has been reported, but a single case of complete heart block with subsequent fetal death has been reported when the drug was combined with digoxin. Verapamil is excreted in human milk, giving rise to the potential for adverse reactions in infants. This fact is of greater concern with the high doses necessary for the management of cluster headache, for which there are no data.

Nifedipine has been associated with cardiovascular defects in first-trimester exposure and with growth retardation in the second and third trimesters. However, it is compatible with breast feeding.

Angiotensin II receptor antagonists

Case reports have described congenital malformations, fetal renal damage, oligohydramnios, skull effects, and death in infants exposed to angiotensin II receptor antagonists in utero. There are no data on excretion into human milk.

Angiotension-converting enzyme inhibitors

Lisinopril is used for migraine prophylaxis. In common with other angiotension-converting enzyme inhibitors, it poses no significant fetal risk during the first trimester. During the second and third trimesters it is toxic and teratogenic, causing prematurity, intrauterine growth retardation, renal tubular dysplasia, severe oligohydramnios leading to fetal distress, lung hypoplasia, skull hypoplasia, limb contractures, neonatal hypotension, and anuria. It is not known whether this drug is excreted in human milk.

Antiepileptics

Gabapentin This drug has been used in early pregnancy for epilepsy without evidence of harm. Gabapentin is secreted into human milk following oral administration with a maximum dose exposure of approximately 1 mg/kg/d.

Topiramate There have been reports of increased risk of oral clefts following exposure to topiramate in pregnancy. Relatively low levels are excreted into human milk.

Valproic acid There is a high risk of fetal abnormalities following exposure to valproic acid during pregnancy. The concentration of valproic acid in breast milk is very low.

Botulinum toxin

There are no human data regarding teratogenicity or excretion into breast milk.

Lithium

Exposure to therapeutic doses of lithium in pregnancy can cause teratogenic and other toxic effects in the fetus and neonate. Maternal thyroid should be monitored and supplementation provided and, if necessary, neonatal thyroid function should also be monitored. There are conflicting opinions as to whether lithium should be stopped during the first trimester of pregnancy and restarted in the second trimester.

During delivery, renal clearance of lithium decreases with the potential for toxicity in the mother and the neonate. Neonatal toxicity may result in hypotonia, cyanosis, goiter, hypothyroidism, poor thermoregulation, and low Apgar scores in the neonate. A floppy infant syndrome has been described. A detailed ultrasound scan and a detailed fetal echocardiography should be offered at around 20 weeks' gestation in all women on lithium therapy. The dose of lithium, if clinically possible, should be reduced near term or discontinued to reduce the risk of neonatal toxicity. Lithium is excreted in breast milk and has been associated with adverse effects in the infant.

Methysergide

Methysergide has been withdrawn in the United States but is still available in other countries. As with other ergot alkaloids, methysergide has significant potential adverse effects on pregnancy and breastfeeding.

EMERGENCY TREATMENT OF HEADACHE

Magnesium is used during pregnancy for the management of preeclampsia and can also be used to treat migraine. Intravenous magnesium sulfate, 1 g given intravenously over 15 minutes, was well tolerated and effective in a randomized, single-blind, placebo-controlled trial of 30 patients with migraine.[73] A combination of intravenous prochlorperazine, 10 mg 8-hourly together with intravenous magnesium sulfate, 1 g 12-hourly, was used successfully to abort 2 cases of prolonged migraine aura during pregnancy.[74]

Corticosteroids successfully treat intractable nausea and vomiting in hyperemesis gravidarum. A 6-day reducing course of prednisolone (60 mg/d for 2 days, 40 mg/d for 2 days, and 20 mg/d for 2 days) can be considered to treat long-duration attacks, particularly if there is evidence of medication overuse.[75] Chronic exposure to high doses of steroids in pregnancy should be avoided because it may cause fetal/neonatal adrenal suppression, and increased incidence of congenital anomalies, neonatal cataract, and stillbirth have been reported when the drug was used throughout pregnancy. Prednisone/prednisolone is compatible with breastfeeding.

SUMMARY

Primary headaches, particularly migraine, are affected by the hormonal changes during pregnancy and lactation. The headaches pose no threat to the pregnancy, so it is important that treatment is equally benign. However, women with migraine should be carefully monitored during pregnancy because they are at increased risk of hypertensive disorders of pregnancy and stroke. Most drugs used to treat headaches can be continued throughout pregnancy. Aspirin and NSAIDs are safe in the first and second trimesters but should be avoided near term. NSAIDs, with the exception of aspirin, can be used during lactation. Women who have taken triptans in the first trimester can be reassured that their use is unlikely to affect the pregnancy. If triptans are indicated during pregnancy and lactation, sumatriptan is the triptan of choice. Ergots are contraindicated. Oxygen can be continued for acute treatment of cluster headache. If prophylaxis is necessary, propranolol is the drug of choice during pregnancy and lactation. Amitriptyline can be used during the first and second trimester of pregnancy and during lactation. Verapamil is indicated for prophylaxis of cluster headache, at the lowest effective doses. Breastfeeding is encouraged for women whose headaches improve during pregnancy, as it sustains the benefits of pregnancy.

RESOURCES

National Library of Medicine Developmental and Reproductive Toxicology Database (DART)
   References to literature on developmental and reproductive toxicology.
   Website: http://toxnet.nlm.nih.gov

National Library of Medicine Drugs and Lactation Database (LactMed)
   A peer-reviewed and fully referenced database of drugs to which breastfeeding mothers may be exposed. Among the data included are maternal and infant levels of drugs, possible effects on breastfed infants and on lactation, and alternative drugs to consider.
   Website: http://toxnet.nlm.nih.gov

Organization of Teratology Information Specialists (OTIS)
   Website: www.OTISpregnancy.org
   Tel.: +1 866 626 6847

Teratogen Information Service (TERIS)
   Website: http://depts.washington.edu/terisweb/teris/

UK Teratology Information Service
   Website: www.toxbase.org
   Tel.: 0844 892 0909 (UK only)

CASE STUDY

V.S., a 34-year-old lawyer, is 12 weeks pregnant with her first child. She had a miscarriage 18 months ago, at 9 weeks. She had migraine without aura since the age of 11 years. Initially she only had occasional attacks, but over the last year she was having an attack twice a month that did not always respond to sumatriptan. She was started on amitriptyline, 50 mg 5 months ago, which reduced the frequency to 1 attack every 4 to 6 weeks, which she could then control with sumatriptan. She stopped the amitriptyline 8 weeks ago, as soon as she realized that she was pregnant. So far during her pregnancy she had 3 migraine attacks, which she treated with an acetaminophen and codeine combination, as she was told that this was the only treatment she could take. This regimen was not effective, and she has already lost 6 days from work through migraine. She is concerned that any medication may increase her chances of another miscarriage but is equally worried that she will not be able to continue work. Other than mild pregnancy-related nausea in the mornings, she is otherwise fit and well and takes no regular medication.

Comment. It is important to reassure V.S. that migraine does not have any adverse effect on the outcome of pregnancy and neither do most medications, including amitriptyline. The doctor stresses the importance of regular snacks and hydration to help migraine and the morning nausea, and suggests more effective options for treating the symptoms of her attacks, noting that because drugs are not licensed for use in pregnancy does not necessarily mean that they will be harmful to the pregnancy. After discussion of the risks and benefits, V.S. decides to try a combination of an NSAID and an antiemetic, understanding that she can use this until the 30th week of pregnancy. She feels relieved that she has the option of taking sumatriptan if necessary. Having understood that the attacks may settle as she enters the second trimester of pregnancy, she feels that she does not need to take a preventive treatment but has the option to return to amitriptyline if the frequency of attacks does not settle. At her review appointment 6 weeks later, V.S. reports that she had one further attack at 11 weeks of pregnancy and has not had any for the last 4 weeks. She agrees to contact the doctor if she has any problems.

REFERENCES

1. Stovner L, Hagen K, Jensen R, et al. The global burden of headache: a documentation of headache prevalence and disability worldwide. Cephalalgia 2007;27(3): 193–210.
2. Cohen AS, Matharu MS, Goadsby PJ. Trigeminal autonomic cephalalgias: current and future treatments. Headache 2007;47(6):969–80.
3. Bahra A, May A, Goadsby PJ. Cluster headache: a prospective clinical study with diagnostic implications. Neurology 2002;58(3):354–61.
4. Cripe SM, Frederick IO, Qiu C, et al. Risk of preterm delivery and hypertensive disorders of pregnancy in relation to maternal co-morbid mood and migraine disorders during pregnancy. Paediatr Perinat Epidemiol 2011;25(2):116–23.
5. Finer LB, Henshaw SK. Disparities in rates of unintended pregnancy in the United States, 1994 and 2001. Perspect Sex Reprod Health 2006;38(2):90–6.
6. Rasmussen BK. Migraine and tension-type headache in a general population: precipitating factors, female hormones, sleep pattern and relation to lifestyle. Pain 1993;53(1):65–72.
7. Maggioni F, Alessi C, Maggino T, et al. Headache during pregnancy. Cephalalgia 1997;17(7):765–9.

8. Ertresvag JM, Zwart JA, Helde G, et al. Headache and transient focal neurological symptoms during pregnancy, a prospective cohort. Acta Neurol Scand 2005; 111(4):233–7.

9. Aegidius K, Zwart JA, Hagen K, et al. The effect of pregnancy and parity on headache prevalence: the Head-HUNT study. Headache 2009;49(6):851–9.

10. Ekbom K, Waldenlind E. Cluster headache in women: evidence of hypofertility(?) Headaches in relation to menstruation and pregnancy. Cephalalgia 1981;1(3): 167–74.

11. van Vliet JA, Favier I, Helmerhorst FM, et al. Cluster headache in women: relation with menstruation, use of oral contraceptives, pregnancy, and menopause. J Neurol Neurosurg Psychiatry 2006;77(5):690–2.

12. MacGregor EA, Frith A, Ellis J, et al. Incidence of migraine relative to menstrual cycle phases of rising and falling estrogen. Neurology 2006;67:2154–8.

13. MacGregor EA, Frith A, Ellis J, et al. Prevention of menstrual attacks of migraine: a double-blind placebo-controlled crossover study. Neurology 2006;67:2159–63.

14. MacGregor EA. Oestrogen and attacks of migraine with and without aura. Lancet Neurol 2004;3(6):354–61.

15. Lance J, Anthony M. Some clinical aspects of migraine. Arch Neurol 1966;15: 356–61.

16. Somerville BW. A study of migraine in pregnancy. Neurology 1972;22(8):824–8.

17. Manzoni GC, Farina S, Granella F, et al. Classic and common migraine suggestive clinical evidence of two separate entities. Funct Neurol 1986;1(2):112–22.

18. Ratinahirana H, Darbois Y, Bousser MG. Migraine and pregnancy: a prospective study in 703 women after delivery. Neurology 1990;40(Suppl 1):437.

19. Rasmussen BK, Olesen J. Migraine with aura and migraine without aura: an epidemiological study. Cephalalgia 1992;12(4):221–8.

20. Granella F, Sances G, Zanferrari C, et al. Migraine without aura and reproductive life events: a clinical epidemiological study in 1300 women. Headache 1993; 33(7):385–9.

21. Cupini LM, Matteis M, Troisi E, et al. Sex-hormone-related events in migrainous females. A clinical comparative study between migraine with aura and migraine without aura. Cephalalgia 1995;15(2):140–4.

22. Russell MB, Rasmussen BK, Fenger K, et al. Migraine without aura and migraine with aura are distinct clinical entities: a study of four hundred and eighty-four male and female migraineurs from the general population. Cephalalgia 1996; 16(4):239–45.

23. MacGregor EA, Igarashi H, Wilkinson M. Headaches and hormones: subjective versus objective assessment. Headache Q 1997;8:126–36.

24. Bille B. A 40-year follow-up of school children with migraine. Cephalalgia 1997; 17:488–91.

25. Mattsson P, Svardsudd K, Lundberg PO, et al. The prevalence of migraine in women aged 40-74 years: a population-based study. Cephalalgia 2000;20(10):893–9.

26. Granella F, Sances G, Pucci E, et al. Migraine with aura and reproductive life events: a case control study. Cephalalgia 2000;20(8):701–7.

27. Kelman L. Women's issues of migraine in tertiary care. Headache 2004;44(1):2–7.

28. Chen TC, Leviton A. Headache recurrence in pregnant women with migraine. Headache 1994;34:107–10.

29. Scharff L, Marcus DA, Turk DC. Headache during pregnancy and in the postpartum: a prospective study. Headache 1997;37(4):203–10.

30. Marcus DA, Scharff L, Turk D. Longitudinal prospective study of headache during pregnancy and postpartum. Headache 1999;39(9):625–32.

31. Sances G, Granella F, Nappi RE, et al. Course of migraine during pregnancy and postpartum: a prospective study. Cephalalgia 2003;23(3):197–205.
32. Melhado E, Maciel JA Jr, Guerreiro CA. Headaches during pregnancy in women with a prior history of menstrual headaches. Arq Neuropsiquiatr 2005;63(4):934–40.
33. Kvisvik EV, Stovner LJ, Helde G, et al. Headache and migraine during pregnancy and puerperium: the MIGRA-study. J Headache Pain 2011;12(4):443–51.
34. Chancellor AM, Wroe SJ, Cull RE. Migraine occurring for the first time in pregnancy. Headache 1990;30(4):224–7.
35. Ertresvag JM, Stovner LJ, Kvavik LE, et al. Migraine aura or transient ischemic attacks? A five-year follow-up case-control study of women with transient central nervous system disorders in pregnancy. BMC Med 2007;5:19.
36. Liberman A, Karussis D, Ben-Hur T, et al. Natural course and pathogenesis of transient focal neurologic symptoms during pregnancy. Arch Neurol 2008; 65(2):218–20.
37. Mandel S. Hemiplegic migraine in pregnancy. Headache 1988;28:414–6.
38. Stein G, Morton J, Marsh A, et al. Headaches after childbirth. Acta Neurol Scand 1984;69(2):74–9.
39. Saurel-Cubizolles MJ, Romito P, Lelong N, et al. Women's health after childbirth: a longitudinal study in France and Italy. BJOG 2000;107(10):1202–9.
40. Goldszmidt E, Kern R, Chaput A, et al. The incidence and etiology of postpartum headaches: a prospective cohort study. Can J Anaesth 2005;52(9):971–7.
41. Campbell OM, Gray RH. Characteristics and determinants of postpartum ovarian function in women in the United States. Am J Obstet Gynecol 1993;169:55–60.
42. Wainscott G, Sullivan M, Volans G, et al. The outcome of pregnancy in women suffering from migraine. Postgrad Med 1978;54:98–102.
43. Banhidy F, Acs N, Horvath-Puho E, et al. Maternal severe migraine and risk of congenital limb deficiencies. Birth Defects Res A Clin Mol Teratol 2006;76(8): 592–601.
44. Chen HM, Chen SF, Chen YH, et al. Increased risk of adverse pregnancy outcomes for women with migraines: a nationwide population-based study. Cephalalgia 2010;30(4):433–8.
45. Olesen C, Steffensen FH, Sorensen HT, et al. Pregnancy outcome following prescription for sumatriptan. Headache 2000;40(1):20–4.
46. Banhidy F, Acs N, Horvath-Puho E, et al. Pregnancy complications and delivery outcomes in pregnant women with severe migraine. Eur J Obstet Gynecol Reprod Biol 2007;134(2):157–63.
47. Rotton WN, Sachtleben MR, Friedman EA. Migraine and eclampsia. Obstet Gynecol 1959;14:322–30.
48. Adeney KL, Williams MA, Miller RS, et al. Risk of preeclampsia in relation to maternal history of migraine headaches. J Matern Fetal Neonatal Med 2005; 18(3):167–72.
49. Davie CA, O'Brien P. Stroke and pregnancy. J Neurol Neurosurg Psychiatry 2008; 79(3):240–5.
50. James AH, Bushnell CD, Jamison MG, et al. Incidence and risk factors for stroke in pregnancy and the puerperium. Obstet Gynecol 2005;106(3):509–16.
51. Von Wald T, Walling AD. Headache during pregnancy. Obstet Gynecol Surv 2002; 57(3):179–85.
52. ACOG. ACOG Committee Opinion #299: guidelines for diagnostic imaging during pregnancy. Obstet Gynecol 2004;104(3):647.
53. Webb JA, Thomsen HS, Morcos SK. The use of iodinated and gadolinium contrast media during pregnancy and lactation. Eur Radiol 2005;15(6):1234–40.

54. Martin PR, MacLeod C. Behavioral management of headache triggers: avoidance of triggers is an inadequate strategy. Clin Psychol Rev 2009;29(6):483–95.
55. Rasmussen BK. Migraine and tension-type headache in a general population: psychosocial factors. Int J Epidemiol 1992;21(6):1138–43.
56. Nestoriuc Y, Rief W, Martin A. Meta-analysis of biofeedback for tension-type headache: efficacy, specificity, and treatment moderators. J Consult Clin Psychol 2008;76(3):379–96.
57. Marcus DA, Scharff L, Turk DC. Nonpharmacological management of headaches during pregnancy. Psychosom Med 1995;57(6):527–35.
58. Scharff L, Marcus DA, Turk DC. Maintenance of effects in the nonmedical treatment of headaches during pregnancy. Headache 1996;36(5):285–90.
59. Linde K, Allais G, Brinkhaus B, et al. Acupuncture for tension-type headache. Cochrane Database Syst Rev 2009;1:CD007587.
60. Linde K, Allais G, Brinkhaus B, et al. Acupuncture for migraine prophylaxis. Cochrane Database Syst Rev 2009;1:CD001218.
61. Neri I, Allais G, Schiapparelli P, et al. Acupuncture versus pharmacological approach to reduce hyperemesis gravidarum discomfort. Minerva Ginecol 2005;57(4):471–5.
62. Sandor PS, Di Clemente L, Coppola G, et al. Efficacy of coenzyme Q10 in migraine prophylaxis: a randomized controlled trial. Neurology 2005;64(4):713–5.
63. Teran E, Hernandez I, Nieto B, et al. Coenzyme Q10 supplementation during pregnancy reduces the risk of pre-eclampsia. Int J Gynaecol Obstet 2009; 105(1):43–5.
64. Evers S, Áfra J, Frese A, et al. EFNS guideline on the drug treatment of migraine: revised report of an EFNS task force. Eur J Neurol 2009;16:968–81.
65. Altman D, Carroli G, Duley L, et al. Do women with pre-eclampsia, and their babies, benefit from magnesium sulphate? The Magpie Trial: a randomised placebo-controlled trial. Lancet 2002;359(9321):1877–90.
66. Nezvalová-Henriksen K, Spigset O, Nordeng H. Triptan exposure during pregnancy and the risk of major congenital malformations and adverse pregnancy outcomes: results from the Norwegian Mother and Child Cohort Study. Headache 2010;50(4):563–75.
67. Bendtsen L, Evers S, Linde M, et al. EFNS guideline on the treatment of tension-type headache—report of an EFNS task force. Eur J Neurol 2010;17(11):1318–25.
68. Jüergens TP, Schaefer C, May A. Treatment of cluster headache in pregnancy and lactation. Cephalalgia 2009;29(4):391–400.
69. The National Teratology Information Service. Hyperbaric oxygen exposure in pregnancy. 2006. Available at: http://www.toxbase.org/. Accessed September 1, 2011.
70. Wojnar-Horton RE, Hackett LP, Yapp P, et al. Distribution and excretion of sumatriptan in human milk. Br J Clin Pharmacol 1996;41(3):217–21.
71. American Academy of Pediatrics. The transfer of drugs and other chemicals into human milk. Pediatrics 2001;108:776–89.
72. Nelson-Piercy C, De Swiet M. Letter: low dose aspirin may be used for prophylaxis. BMJ 1996;313(7058):691.
73. Demirkaya S, Vural O, Dora B, et al. Efficacy of intravenous magnesium sulfate in the treatment of acute migraine attacks. Headache 2001;41(2):171–7.
74. Rozen TD. Aborting a prolonged migrainous aura with intravenous prochlorperazine and magnesium sulfate. Headache 2003;43(8):901–3.
75. Krymchantowski AV, Barbosa JS. Prednisone as initial treatment of analgesic-induced daily headache. Cephalalgia 2000;20:107–13.

76. Moore MP, Redman CW. Case-control study of severe pre-eclampsia of early onset. Br Med J (Clin Res Ed) 1983;287(6392):580–3.
77. Marcoux S, Berube S, Brisson J, et al. History of migraine and risk of pregnancy-induced hypertension. Epidemiology 1992;3(1):53–6.
78. Facchinetti F, Allais G, D'Amico R, et al. The relationship between headache and preeclampsia: a case-control study. Eur J Obstet Gynecol Reprod Biol 2005; 121(2):143–8.
79. Scher AI, Terwindt GM, Picavet HS, et al. Cardiovascular risk factors and migraine: the GEM population-based study. Neurology 2005;64(4):614–20.
80. Facchinetti F, Allais G, Nappi R, et al. Migraine is a risk factor for hypertensive disorders in pregnancy: a prospective cohort study. Cephalalgia 2009;29(3): 286–92.
81. Sanchez SE, Qiu C, Williams MA, et al. Headaches and migraines are associated with an increased risk of preeclampsia in Peruvian women. Am J Hypertens 2008; 21(3):360–4.

The Postpartum Period in Women with Epilepsy

Autumn Klein, MD, PhD

KEYWORDS

- Postpartum • Epilepsy • Breastfeeding • Depression • Antiepileptic medications
- Pregnancy • Women

KEY POINTS

- Breastfeeding is encouraged in women with epilepsy (WWE).
- WWE are concerned about caring for their newborn infant. Advanced planning can decrease the risk of injury to mother and newborn.
- WWE are at increased risk of postpartum depression. Early awareness can lead to faster treatment.
- Discuss postpartum contraception during pregnancy.

CASE

L.M. is a 30 year-old left-handed woman with juvenile myoclonic epilepsy who was well controlled on valproic acid for many years, but who transitioned to levetiracetam at 28 years of age when she planned to have children. She did well throughout her pregnancy on increasing doses of levetiracetam, with only one event of myoclonus at approximately 6 months of pregnancy, involving a subtherapeutic serum level of levetiracetam in the setting of a delayed dose. Her delivery was uneventful and she started full breastfeeding immediately after. The levetiracetam was lowered at birth to her prepregnancy level with an additional extra 500 mg per day. The baby was healthy and met all developmental milestones with no noted adverse effects from breastfeeding. L.M. would pump an extra few bottles during the day, and her husband would feed the baby once at night. She continued full breastfeeding until the baby was 6 months old, at which time she decreased breastfeeding to 2 times a day.

Disclosure Statement: Dr Klein is a prior EEG consultant for Digitrace, and receives funding from the American Epilepsy Foundation and Epilepsy Foundation of America.
Division of Women's Neurology, Department of Neurology and Obstetrics and Gynecology, UPMC Presbyterian/Magee Womens Hospital of UPMC, University of Pittsburgh, 3471 Fifth Avenue, Suite 811, Pittsburgh, PA 15213, USA
E-mail address: kleinam2@upmc.edu

Neurol Clin 30 (2012) 867–875
http://dx.doi.org/10.1016/j.ncl.2012.06.001
0733-8619/12/$ – see front matter © 2012 Elsevier Inc. All rights reserved.

neurologic.theclinics.com

BREASTFEEDING

Breastfeeding is gaining popularity in the United States, but rates are still low for a developed country. The 2011 Breastfeeding Report Card showed that in the United States, overall 74.6% of women have ever breastfed, with only 35% and 14.8% of women, respectively, exclusively breastfeeding at 3 and 6 months.[1] In one recent study whose participants were largely educated Caucasian women, 42% of women with epilepsy (WWE) studied were breastfeeding.[2]

Breastfeeding has many short-term and long-term health benefits for mothers as well as for infant health, immunity, growth, and development.[3,4] Breastfeeding decreases a woman's risk of developing diabetes, breast cancer, and ovarian cancer, and in infants it reduces the risk of ear infections, asthma, diarrheal illnesses, obesity, leukemia, and sudden infant death syndrome.[3] It is also psychologically beneficial to both mother and child, and promotes mother-infant attachment.

Psychosocial Concern

Many WWE are hesitant to breastfeed their children, the reasons for which are not well understood. Influential factors include psychosocial situation, disease severity, anti-epileptic medication, the effects of breastfeeding on seizures, and the effects of seizures on breastfeeding. Some WWE believe that the amount of medication their offspring experiences in breast milk is more than the amount of medication exposure in utero. Many WWE view antiepileptic drug (AED) exposure through breast milk as voluntary, and avoid breastfeeding to minimize the potential for further exposure. In general, however, the child experiences less medication through breastfeeding than when in utero.

Psychosocial factors, including a mother's initial determination to breastfeed, the amount of time with the child, and the personal support from her family, workplace, and health care system, determine whether a mother will breastfeed. Breastfeeding can be challenging for many women to begin, and often requires education and direction. If a lactation consultant is not available, breastfeeding instruction is limited to nursing staff. If a child is premature or has trouble latching and suckling, or if the child has experienced medications in utero that may make him or her more lethargic for the first few days, breastfeeding is more difficult to initiate. After discharge from the hospital, many women have no instruction unless someone is hired to come into the home.

Pharmacokinetics

The amount of drug that is excreted into breast milk is dependent on many factors, including the drug's chemical properties, the concentration of the drug in the mother's serum, the mother's metabolism, and the composition of the breast milk itself. Breast milk composition changes over time. Colostrum, which is excreted the first few days postpartum until mature milk comes in, has a high antibody content and relatively more protein and less fat than later, more mature milk. Mature milk is composed of foremilk, which is more watery and less fat laden than the later hindmilk.

Properties of the drug that determine its secretion into breast milk include its molecular weight, protein binding, and lipophilicity. The lower the molecular weight, the less the protein binding and the higher the lipophilicity, make it more likely for the drug to be excreted into breast milk. The ionization of the drug also plays a role in whether the drug is excreted into breast milk such that cationic or basic drugs will be excreted into the milk. Pharmacokinetics of drugs are altered in pregnancy and postpartum and do not return to a prepregnancy state for up to 3 months postpartum, making drug secretion into the breast milk dynamic over time. Other factors that are more difficult to determine are the time from administration of drug to breastfeeding, the frequency of dosing, the frequency of breastfeeding, and the duration of breastfeeding. Reported levels typically are only from one sample, but ideally multiple samples are needed to assess an accurate level of medication in breast milk.

Drug levels can be measured in breast milk, but this does not correlate with what the child is absorbing or experiencing. Newborns are inefficient at extracting medication from breast milk and their ability to metabolize and excrete medications is immature, potentially leading to an accumulation of drug absorbed. There are several ways to estimate the amount of drug in breast milk or in the child, none of which is perfectly accurate.

The most common way to measure the amount of drug in breast milk is the milk-to-plasma (MP) ratio, which can be determined by directly sampling breast milk or by using a calculation that takes the chemical properties of the drug into account. If the MP ratio is greater than 1, the drug is thought to be concentrated in breast milk, although. This ratio does not always relate to the infant serum level, which can be directly measured by serum samples from the child, or can be calculated. The infant dose, which is a measurement of the amount of drug from breast milk to which the child is exposed, is determined by the concentration of drug in breast milk multiplied by the volume of breast milk consumed by the child each day. Both the amount of drug in breast milk and the amount of breast milk ingested by a child can be difficult to determine accurately, so these numbers should be interpreted with caution. Alternatively, a maternal weight-adjusted infant dose can be calculated by using the infant dose and adjusting for maternal serum dose and maternal weight.

Finally, infant drug clearance is a factor that determines drug concentration in the child. Compared with adults, newborns have immature liver enzymes and slowed renal excretion, leading to potential drug accumulation. In children who are born premature or small for gestational age, these metabolic pathways may be even more immature. Depending on the pathway, some of these processes may not reach adult levels for several years.

Newborns are known to withdraw from opiates, but a definitive AED withdrawal syndrome is not known. There are rare reports of newborn behaviors that have been interpreted as withdrawal (see later section on drugs). Symptoms that have been reported are sedation, lethargy, irritability, excessive crying, altered sleep patterns, vomiting, difficulty feeding, and tremor. Children born to mothers taking high-dose barbiturates, such as primidone or phenobarbital, and benzodiazepines are potentially vulnerable to withdrawal and may need observation, but this should be evaluated on a case-by-case basis. One case report suggested that breastfeeding may minimize withdrawal symptoms, suggesting that over time the child experiences less medication.[5] There are few criteria for withdrawal in neonates, and there is usually greater scrutiny in offspring of WWE, biasing observation of potential withdrawal symptoms.

Newborn serum drug levels are the most accurate way to assess drug effects, and if necessary this can be done by heelstick to minimize the child's discomfort. One measurement may not accurately reflect the overall exposure, so if there are continued concerns over behavior or symptoms, more levels can be measured. Adverse effects of drugs from breast milk are most commonly reported in children younger than 6 months, which coincides with when many women breastfeed. In a large study of almost 900 women taking medications while breastfeeding, only 10% reported minor effects in the child, but none were medically significant.[6] The serum level at which clinical effects occur for drugs ingested through breast milk is unknown. Many drugs being taken by breastfeeding mothers are not used routinely enough for direct effects and levels in newborns to be known. Based on a study of different classes of drugs, including antiepileptics, when the infant's serum level is less than 10% of the mother's serum level standardized by weight, or less than 10% of the infant serum level if therapeutic levels are known in the infant, it is considered clinically insignificant.[6] If levels are higher, risks and benefits should be discussed with the patient, but most women can still continue to breastfeed with careful monitoring of the child. The maturity of newborns' metabolism also determines their serum drug level.

The UDP-glucuronyltransferase enzymes, which metabolize lamotrigine (LTG) and some hormones, do not increase to the adult levels until about 20 months of age.[7] There is only one reported case of possible LTG toxicity in an infant who had apnea,[8] but in general LTG is thought to be well tolerated in breastfeeding infants. Similarly, renal clearance is slowed at birth but reaches nearly adult levels within months. Genetic polymorphisms and other factors that affect drug metabolism have not been well studied in infants.

POSTPARTUM DRUG DOSE ADJUSTMENT

During pregnancy, many AEDs are adjusted upwards to overcome the increase in drug metabolism and/or clearance that occurs in pregnancy. There is an increase in renal blood flow by 100%, so that renally cleared drugs, such as levetiracetam (LVT), show a 50% decrease in serum level during pregnancy if no dose changes are made.[9] The rate of glucuronidation of drugs is increased in pregnancy under the influence of estrogens, such that drugs like LTG that use this pathway have an increased clearance in pregnancy.[10] Many epileptologists adjust LTG throughout pregnancy to maintain a baseline level that correlates with good seizure control before pregnancy. A recent algorithm suggested LTG adjustments in pregnancy and postpartum.[11] For many other AEDs, doses are increased throughout pregnancy to maintain a therapeutic serum level, but they often do not need changes as drastic as those needed with LTG. In making these adjustments, many women are at higher doses of AEDs at the time of delivery compared with prepregnancy. As renal and hepatic clearance return to prepregnancy levels within the weeks to months after delivery, many women may become overmedicated or toxic if there is no postpartum decrease in the AED dose. There is no consensus on how to adjust medications postpartum, but there are several options: no adjustment, wait until WWE complains of overmedicated symptoms and then adjust downward, or adjust medications back to prepregnancy doses (or close to those doses) at the time of delivery or shortly thereafter.

Antiepileptic Drugs

The American Academy of Neurology (AAN) and the American Academy of Pediatrics (AAP) have published guidelines on AEDs and breastfeeding to provide direction for management for patients and physicians. The AAN practice parameters concluded that primidone (PRM) and LVT penetrate into breast milk in potentially clinically important amounts.[12] The AAN also noted that valproate (VPA), phenobarbital, phenytoin (PHT), and carbamazepine (CBZ) probably do not pass into the breast milk in clinically significant quantities, and gabapentin, LTG, and topiramate possibly pass into breast milk in potentially clinically significant amounts. Their final statement was that "the clinical consequences for the newborn of ingesting AEDs via breast milk remain sorely underexplored and will continue to produce anxiety in WWE bearing children and all who care for these clinical dyads."[12] It is generally believed that the benefits of lactation outweigh the risks of AED exposure despite the lack of information on AEDs in breast milk.

Balancing the risks and benefits of breastfeeding needs careful consideration in WWE who are taking barbiturates and benzodiazepines. Levels of phenobarbital and primidone are low in breast milk, but it is generally not recommended to breast-feed while taking these drugs. It has been shown that serum levels in the newborn are higher than in the serum of WWE, and some children have been reported to be sedated.[13] Children breastfed while the mother was taking diazepam have also been noted to have lethargy, weight loss, and sedation. The AAP suggests breastfeed-ing with caution when the mother is taking these drugs.[14]

Most medications are excreted into the breast milk in low amounts, particularly those with higher protein binding such as CBZ, PHT, and VPA. It is for this reason that the AAP suggests that these AEDs are compatible with lactation.[14] Overall, there are very few reports of AED levels in breast milk and infant serum, even for the older AEDs. What is known is presented here.

Valproic acid

An older study using mass spectroscopy to analyze 36 breast-milk samples in 16 patients showed that the VPA levels were very low, at 0.4 to 3.9 µg/mL (mean 1.9 ± 1.2 µg/mL).[15] Six infants exposed to VPA in breast milk were shown to have a serum level 0.9% to 2.3% of the mother's serum level.[16] There is only one known adverse report of an infant who had thrombocytopenia and anemia while being breastfed on VPA, and these abnormalities disappeared when breastfeeding was stopped.[17] Overall, however, valproic acid is considered compatible with breastfeed-ing because of its high protein binding and low excretion in breast milk.

Phenytoin

Similar to VPA, PHT is considered compatible with breastfeeding because of its high protein binding and minimal excretion into breast milk. There have been no recent studies on the levels of PHT in breast milk, but there is a potential accumulation of PHT in the newborn that is due to variability in their metabolism. It has been shown that in infants of mothers taking PHT there are very low levels (<5% of maternal serum) of PHT in the serum,[18] which is thus considered compatible with breastfeeding. There is one report, from 1954, of methemoglobinemia, drowsiness, and decreased suck in one infant breastfed on PHT.[19]

Carbamazepine

An older study showed that the CBZ concentration in breast milk was 36.4% of the maternal serum level, but the infant serum level was not measured.[20] Levels of carba-mazepine are low in breast milk, and milk/maternal serum levels in 2 pregnancies were found to be 0.64 and 0.3.[21] The only reported adverse effects of CBZ in breastfeeding were liver dysfunction and hepatitis.[22]

Lamotrigine

The largest case series of LTG in breast milk studied 210 samples of breast milk from 30 women.[23] The milk to maternal plasma ratio was 41.3%, with an infant serum dose of 18.9% that of the maternal serum dose. The only side effect noted was mild throm-bocytopenia in the infants. Several prior studies had shown similar results.[24] In one case report, a child exposed to LTG through full breastfeeding had an episode of ap-nea, but the level of LTG at the time of the event 16 days after birth was 4.87 µg/mL compared with 7.71 µg/mL 12.5 hours after birth.[8] Even though glucuronidation path-ways in children are not fully developed until they are several years old, these studies suggest that LTG is not accumulating in the children.

Levetiracetam

In one study of 11 mothers taking LVT who gave breast milk and infant serum samples, the average milk/maternal serum ratio was 1.05 (range 0.78–1.55) and the infant's level was 13% of the mother's serum level,[25] suggesting that the infant absorbs only a small amount. Another study followed 8 mothers and their infants from birth to 10 months of age.[26] At 3 to 5 days, milk/maternal serum level was 1.00 (range 0.76–1.33) and the infant serum levels were very low at 10 to 15 µM, and all later time points were similar.

Topiramate

Breast-milk information on 5 mother-child pairs showed a milk/maternal plasma ratio of 0.86 (range 0.67–1.1) at 2 to 3 weeks after delivery, and was similar again at 1 and 3 months postpartum.[27] Two to 3 weeks after delivery, infants had barely detectable levels (>0.9 µM) that could not be quantified, and one had undetectable levels. Only one child had diarrhea while the mother was breastfeeding and taking topiramate.

Zonisamide

In 2 mothers taking zonisamade, 41% to 57% of the drug was excreted into the breast milk.[28] There are no reports of adverse events in an infant exposed to zonisamide through breast milk, but studies are limited.

Other AEDs

Infants may accumulate phenobarbital and primidone, so caution is warranted when breastfeeding, and the child should be monitored for adverse effects. There are few reports about clonazepam and clobazam and breastfeeding in the literature, but caution is warranted, and it is recommended to look for sedation. It is suggested not to breastfeed while taking felbamate, given issues with aplastic anemia, but there are no cases reported. Little is known about gabapentin and oxcarbazepine, but there are no adverse effects reported while breastfeeding. There are no known reports of breastfeeding with lacosamide, pregabalin, retigabine, rufinamide, tigabine, or vigabatrin. Although there is no consensus, it would generally not be recommended for a woman to start on an AED postpartum while breastfeeding if the offspring was not exposed to an AED in utero.

COGNITIVE ISSUES

Information on the cognitive and behavioral outcomes of children born to WWE taking AEDs and breastfeeding is limited. In the Neurocognitive Effects of Antiepileptic Drugs (NEAD) study, the IQ of offspring of WWE taking monotherapy of either CBZ, LTG, PHT, or VPA were compared by drug and breastfeeding status.[2] Children breastfed versus those who were not showed no difference in IQ, comparing them either as a group or within each drug group. This finding suggests that breastfeeding may not have an adverse effect on cognition, but more studies need to be done.

SAFETY ISSUES

The safety of mother and child in the setting of seizures is important during pregnancy, and perhaps more so in the postpartum period. Lack of sleep and missed medications can increase a new mother's risk of seizure. In addition, the postpartum period brings physical and emotional challenges that make WWE especially vulnerable during this time. Postpartum safety is usually overlooked in discussions with pregnant WWE, and if a new mother sees her neurologist after delivery, safety is often overshadowed by concerns over seizures and AED management in the postpartum period. Ironically, in a study done in the United Kingdom, WWE were found to be more concerned about the risks of caring for their baby and less about breastfeeding and medication management.[29] Nearly 50% of the women were given information on safety, 86% of whom found it useful.

Sleep deprivation is a feature of the postpartum period for all mothers, but in WWE this is a paramount concern. The planning of situations so that sleep deprivation is avoided in WWE is an important step to prevent seizures, and arranging help from a spouse, family, or hired help is needed. If a mother is breastfeeding, nighttime feedings are usually more frequent, and having someone to help is critical. Breast milk can be pumped during the day to be stored and fed at night so that the WWE can sleep.

Reviewing daily activities and making sure the mother and child are safe should a seizure occur can be done in advance of the delivery. If the mother experiences an aura, placing the child in a crib or seat as soon as the warning starts is suggested.

For the mother with an aura or warning, suggesting that she place the baby in a crib or other enclosed safe space as soon as she gets the warning is suggested. For mothers with jerks from myoclonic seizures, avoiding sleep deprivation and alcohol, or avoiding high-risk times when the myoclonus may occur (eg, in the morning) is the ideal way to avoid the myoclonus.

If the WWE has no warning, for the first few weeks postpartum it is encouraged to consider having another caregiver present. Bathing a child or breastfeeding the child in bed when the mother is alone is not recommended. Any activities, such as changing the baby or playing with the child, are best done as close to the ground as possible in case the mother falls down or lays down during a seizure. Although some of these arrangements may make the WWE feel less independent, the safety of the child should be stressed.

As children get older and start to crawl or walk, keeping them in an enclosed area can reduce the risk of wandering into dangerous situations should the mother have a seizure. If mother and child go outside the home, an emergency plan should be considered in advance. Going to a public place, preferably where those around are aware that the mother has epilepsy, is suggested. Placing a message on or near the child with emergency contact information in case the mother has a seizure can be helpful. Epilepsy support groups where WWE can share safety plans may decrease anxiety for WWE.

DEPRESSION

Postpartum depression (PPD) is characterized by mood swings, irritability, tearfulness, fatigue, and confusion. PPD usually occurs in the first few weeks postpartum, and is often transient. Approximately 15% of women have postpartum depression, but women with prepregnancy depression are at higher risk.[30] Psychotherapy and antidepressants, if needed, are the ideal treatments, but access to psychotherapy in the postpartum period is difficult for many women, and many are reluctant to take medications while breastfeeding.

Two studies have shown that the rates of PPD are higher in WWE compared with the general population.[31,32] In one study, using the Edinburgh Postnatal Depression Scale, it was shown that 29% of WWE had PPD compared with only 11% of the controls.[31] In another study using the Beck Depression Inventory in 56 WWE during pregnancy and postpartum, 25% of women had PPD.[32] PPD was associated with multiparity and AED polytherapy but not a specific AED. WWE have many reasons to be at an increased risk of PPD. WWE have a higher rate of depression than the general population, seizures can interfere with the care of their newborn, and the inability to drive may limit their mobility and social interaction. WWE need support and reassurance from their physician and family during the postpartum period. Discussions during pregnancy and knowing about the increased risks of PPD in WWE can help with awareness and early identification.

CONTRACEPTION IN THE POSTPARTUM PERIOD

Discussing future family planning during pregnancy may prevent unintended pregnancies. Many women still believe that they cannot get pregnant while breastfeeding or during the postpartum period. Although this aspect is beyond the scope of this article, contraception should be discussed with WWE during pregnancy in or at the time of delivery, to avoid delay.

REFERENCES

1. Breastfeeding report card—United States, 2011. Centers for Disease Control and Prevention; 2011. Available at: http://www.cdc.gov/breastfeeding/data/reportcard.htm. Accessed May 29, 2012.
2. Meador KJ, Baker GA, Browning N, et al. Effects of breastfeeding in children of women taking antiepileptic drugs. Neurology 2010;75(22):1954–60.
3. Agency for Healthcare Research and Quality. Breastfeeding and maternal and infant health outcomes in developed countries. Rockville (MD); 2007. Available at: http://www.ahrq.gov/clinic/tp/brfouttp.htm. Accessed June 4, 2012.
4. American Academy of Pediatrics Section on Breastfeeding. Breastfeeding and the use of human milk. Pediatrics 2005;115(2):496–506.
5. Rauchenzauner M, Kiechl-Kohlendorfer U, Rostasy K, et al. Old and new antiepileptic drugs during pregnancy and lactation—report of a case. Epilepsy Behav 2011;20(4):719–20.
6. Ito S. Drug therapy for breast-feeding women. N Engl J Med 2000;343(2):118–26.
7. Miyagi SJ, Collier AC. Pediatric development of glucuronidation: the ontogeny of hepatic UGT1A4. Drug Metab Dispos 2007;35(9):1587–92.
8. Nordmo E, Aronsen L, Wasland K, et al. Severe apnea in an infant exposed to lamotrigine in breast milk. Ann Pharmacother 2009;43(11):1893–7.
9. Tomson T, Battino D. Pharmacokinetics and therapeutic drug monitoring of newer antiepileptic drugs during pregnancy and the puerperium. Clin Pharm 2007;46(3):209–19.
10. Pennell PB. Pregnancy in women who have epilepsy. Neurol Clin 2004;22(4):799–820.
11. Sabers A. Algorithm for lamotrigine dose adjustment before, during, and after pregnancy. Acta Neurol Scand 2012;126(1):e1–4.
12. Harden CL, Pennell PB, Koppel BS, et al. Practice parameter update: management issues for women with epilepsy—focus on pregnancy (an evidence-based review): vitamin K, folic acid, blood levels, and breastfeeding: report of the Quality Standards Subcommittee and Therapeutics and Technology Assessment Subcommittee of the American Academy of Neurology and American Epilepsy Society. Neurology 2009;73(2):142–9.
13. Kaneko S, Sato T, Suzuki K. The levels of anticonvulsants in breast milk. Br J Clin Pharmacol 1979;7(6):624–7.
14. American Academy of Pediatrics Committee on Drugs. Transfer of drugs and other chemicals into human milk. Pediatrics 2001;108(3):776–89.
15. von Unruh GE, Froescher W, Hoffmann F, et al. Valproic acid in breast milk: how much is really there? Ther Drug Monit 1984;6(3):272–6.

16. Piontek CM, Baab S, Peindl KS, et al. Serum valproate levels in 6 breastfeeding mother-infant pairs. J Clin Psychiatry 2000;61(3):170–2.
17. Stahl MM, Neiderud J, Vinge E. Thrombocytopenic purpura and anemia in a breast-fed infant whose mother was treated with valproic acid. J Pediatr 1997;130(6):1001–3.
18. Steen B, Rane A, Lonnerholm G, et al. Phenytoin excretion in human breast milk and plasma levels in nursed infants. Ther Drug Monit 1982;4(4):331–4.
19. Finch E, Lorber J. Methaemoglobinaemia in the newborn probably due to phenytoin excreted in human milk. J Obstet Gynaecol Br Emp 1954;61(6):833–4.
20. Froescher W, Eichelbaum M, Niesen M, et al. Carbamazepine levels in breast milk. Ther Drug Monit 1984;6(3):266–71.
21. Shimoyama R, Ohkubo T, Sugawara K. Monitoring of carbamazepine and carbamazepine 10,11-epoxide in breast milk and plasma by high-performance liquid chromatography. Ann Clin Biochem 2000;37(Pt 2):210–5.
22. Chaudron LH, Jefferson JW. Mood stabilizers during breastfeeding: a review. J Clin Psychiatry 2000;61(2):79–90.
23. Newport DJ, Pennell PB, Calamaras MR, et al. Lamotrigine in breast milk and nursing infants: determination of exposure. Pediatrics 2008;122(1):e223–31.
24. Fotopoulou C, Kretz R, Bauer S, et al. Prospectively assessed changes in lamotrigine-concentration in women with epilepsy during pregnancy, lactation and the neonatal period. Epilepsy Res 2009;85(1):60–4.
25. Tomson T, Palm R, Kallen K, et al. Pharmacokinetics of levetiracetam during pregnancy, delivery, in the neonatal period, and lactation. Epilepsia 2007;48(6):1111–6.
26. Johannessen SI, Helde G, Brodtkorb E. Levetiracetam concentrations in serum and in breast milk at birth and during lactation. Epilepsia 2005;46(5):775–7.
27. Ohman I, Vitols S, Luef G, et al. Topiramate kinetics during delivery, lactation, and in the neonate: preliminary observations. Epilepsia 2002;43(10):1157–60.
28. Kawada K, Itoh S, Kusaka T, et al. Pharmacokinetics of zonisamide in perinatal period. Brain Dev 2002;24(2):95–7.
29. Bagshaw J, Crawford P, Chappell B. Problems that mothers' with epilepsy experience when caring for their children. Seizure 2008;17(1):42–8.
30. Pearlstein T, Howard M, Salisbury A, et al. Postpartum depression. Am J Obstet Gynecol 2009;200(4):357–64.
31. Turner K, Piazzini A, Franza A, et al. Postpartum depression in women with epilepsy versus women without epilepsy. Epilepsy Behav 2006;9(2):293–7.
32. Galanti M, Newport DJ, Pennell PB, et al. Postpartum depression in women with epilepsy: influence of antiepileptic drugs in a prospective study. Epilepsy Behav 2009;16(3):426–30.

Pregnancy and Multiple Sclerosis

P.K. Coyle, MD

KEYWORDS

• Multiple sclerosis • Pregnancy • Gender issues • Relapse

KEY POINTS

• Multiple sclerosis (MS) is not an inherited disease.
• Pregnancy does not worsen prognosis in MS.
• MS disease activity decreases in pregnancy, particularly during the last trimester.
• About 30% of untreated MS patients experience a relapse 3 months after delivery.
• MS patients can expect normal fertility rates and pregnancy results.

CASE

This 25-year-old woman was just diagnosed and treated for optic neuritis, with excellent recovery. Magnetic resonance imaging (MRI) of her brain and spinal cord, and spinal fluid, are abnormal, consistent with multiple sclerosis (MS). She meets criteria for a diagnosis of MS as outlined by the 2010 McDonald criteria. She is a newlywed, married only 6 months earlier.

Discussion

This woman is a prototypic MS patient, identified at the time of her first relapse. As a recently married young woman, this diagnosis of a treatable but (as yet) incurable neurologic disease raises many issues. She wants to know whether MS will affect her ability to conceive. She wants to know whether she should get pregnant right away, or wait and focus on treating her MS. She worries that she can pass MS on to her child. She also worries about what to expect during and after future pregnancies. There is very good information and advice that can be provided to this MS patient, which is covered in this article.

Financial disclosures: Dr Coyle has received honoraria for educational, consultative, or research funding related to multiple sclerosis from the following companies: Acorda, Actelion, Avanir, Bayer, Biogen, Idec, EMD Serono, Novartis, Questcor, Roche, Sanofi Aventis, and Teva Neurosciences.
Department of Neurology, Stony Brook MS Comprehensive Care Center, Stony Brook University, HSC T-12, Room 020, Stony Brook, NY 11794-8121, USA
E-mail address: patricia.coyle@stonybrookmedicine.edu

Neurol Clin 30 (2012) 877–888
doi:10.1016/j.ncl.2012.05.002
0733-8619/12/$ – see front matter

BACKGROUND

MS is a major neurologic disease with characteristic features (**Box 1**). MS shows a strong female predominance and affects young adults, making the typical patient a young woman of childbearing age. Most individuals (85%) present with relapsing MS, experiencing discrete attacks separated by apparent clinical stability. Untreated patients generally transition to a slowly worsening (progressive) stage. Because there is no meaningful recovery, progressive MS always leads to disability. About 15% of patients present with slow worsening from onset, and are considered to have either primary progressive MS (10%) or progressive relapsing MS (5%). Primary progressive MS patients, by definition, never experience a relapse. If they do, they are reclassified as having progressive relapsing MS. Progressive-from-onset MS presents about a decade later than relapsing MS (late 30s, early 40s), shows an equal gender ratio, and most often involves a gradually worsening myelopathy.

Disease etiology remains unknown, and may be heterogeneous. First, there are genetic factors involved. Nearly 100 associated genes have been identified to date. These genes involve risk/susceptibility, protection, and disease severity.[1]

Second, there are important environmental factors.[2] Implicated factors are vitamin D deficiency, Epstein-Barr virus infection (and particularly when there is clinical expression, mononucleosis), tobacco use, solvent exposure, shift work at a young age, and ultraviolet exposure.[3] With regard to environmental factors and pregnancy, a recent study from Australia reported low maternal exposure to ultraviolet radiation in the first trimester as increasing offspring risk of MS,[4] whereas another study could not show maternal smoking during pregnancy to be a risk factor.[5] Higher milk intake (2–3 glasses)

Box 1
MS characteristic features

- Disease of young adults
  - 90% onset between ages 15 and 50 years
  - Pediatric MS (onset <18 years) 2% to 4%
  - Onset if younger than 10 or older than 60 years is rare (<1%)
- Female predominance
  - 70% to 75% female (except for equal ratio primary progressive MS)
- Variable course
  - Ranges from asymptomatic (autopsy diagnosis) to presymptomatic (radiologically isolated syndrome) to symptomatic
  - Relapsing MS presents as clinically isolated syndrome (85% of MS)
  - Progressive-from-onset MS involves primary progressive (10%), or progressive relapsing (5%)
  - Natural history is for relapsing MS to transition to secondary progressive MS
  - Great individual variability
- More than 90% of patients Caucasian (northern European, Scandinavian background)
- Variable frequency
  - Low-, medium-, high-risk zones
  - Frequency tends to increase moving farther from the equator

during pregnancy and higher maternal vitamin D levels were reported to be associated with lower risk of MS.[6]

Third, MS is an immune-mediated disease with pathologic abnormalities confined to the central nervous system (CNS). The host immune system produces organ-specific abnormality that can include both macroscopic and microscopic injury.[7] Macroscopic plaques involve injury to myelin, axons, oligodendrocytes, and neurons with reactive astrogliosis. These plaques, reflecting focal inflammation, are characteristic of relapsing MS and are visualized very well on MRI. Progressive MS represents clinical expression of the neurodegenerative phase of the disease. Pathology involves microscopic changes including within normal-appearing brain tissue and gray matter, with injury to axons and neurons, microglial activation, and diffuse but low-grade inflammation.

PREGNANCY ISSUES

Pregnancy is a major concern for many MS patients.[8] One study found MS women were somewhat older when they became pregnant.[9] Routine questions that come up, as indicated in the case study, include interactions between MS and pregnancy, fetal risks, genetic implications, how pregnancy affects use of medications, and post-partum management.[10]

Assisted Reproduction Techniques

An early report suggested fertility treatment might increase the risk of relapse when a gonadotropin/luteinizing hormone–releasing hormone agonist was used.[11] A subsequent study of 23 patients suggested that this hormonal stimulation (with either an agonist or antagonist) increased relapses for a 3-month period following the fertility treatment.[12,13] Typically these are patients who are not on therapy, as they are trying to become pregnant.

Prognosis

Up until the 1950s to early 1960s, MS patients were advised not to become pregnant because it would worsen their disease.[14,15] This advice turned out not to be true, and more recent studies indicate that long-term prognosis is more favorable in patients who become pregnant.[16,17] In one study of 200 women, pregnancy was associated with a 6-year delay in wheelchair dependence.[18] In a Belgian study, women with relapsing-from-onset MS and at least 2 pregnancies had reduced disability risk; this association was not found for progressive-from-onset MS.[19] In another hospital-based study of 277 relapsing patients, no association was found between parity and time to secondary progressive disease.[20]

The vast majority of pregnant MS patients have relapsing disease. There has been some concern that progressive MS patients who become pregnant may not do well. However, this remains an anecdotal impression that needs to be investigated.

MS Effect on Pregnancy

For the most part, MS has little to no effect on pregnancy.[21] There is typically no impact on fertility/ability to conceive, pregnancy itself, ability to deliver, or fetal well-being. There is no increase in spontaneous abortions, or major neonatal or obstetric complications.[22] Notable exceptions are that MS can cause sexual dysfunction that may affect libido. A very disabled MS patient who becomes pregnant might require assisted delivery. However, because most pregnant MS patients have relapsing disease and relatively good neurologic examinations, this is rarely an issue. Studies and analyses have reported preterm birth and decreased birth weight in MS babies.[23,24] In a meta-analysis of 22 previous studies published in 2011, 10% of MS deliveries were premature, with decreased birth weight.[21] A recent prospective study from Finland found no impact on birth weight, but reported a greater likelihood of artificial insemination and assisted vaginal delivery.[25] This study was a small one involving 61 MS women. A larger study from British Columbia compared 432 MS births (fewer than 1% of births were to primary progressive MS patients and 4% to secondary progressive) with 2975 control births.[26] There was no difference in mean gestational age, birth weight, assisted vaginal delivery, or cesarean section. MS patients with greater disability did have a slightly increased risk of adverse delivery outcomes.

Pregnancy Effect on MS

Pregnancy involves a shift away from inflammation factors and toward immune tolerance, so the mother will not reject the semiallogeneic fetus. Cell-mediated immunity is downregulated while humoral immunity is enhanced (**Box 2**).[27–38] Multiple immunoregulatory factors are at play during pregnancy, leading to reduced MS activity both clinically and on MRI, which is most marked during the last trimester[39,40]; this is in contradistinction to a disorder such as neuromyelitis optica (Devic disease) whereby attacks may occur during later pregnancy. MS disease onset is unusual during pregnancy.[16] In the Swedish MS register, use of oral contraceptives plus childbirth was associated with a later age of onset of MS.[41] In a much larger Danish cohort, parenthood did not convey protection against MS.[42] Relapses are uncommon during pregnancy. The relapse rate is lowest during the last trimester. Limited data on brain MRI indicate a decrease in silent lesion formation as well. However, in the immediate postpartum period there is a temporary rebound increase in relapse risk that lasts about 12 weeks. Relapse activity then decreases and stays down. Presumably the abrupt change in the immunologic and hormonal milieu is an important factor. In one report a decrease in $CD4^+$ interferon-γ–producing cells postpartum was associated with postpartum relapses.[31]

The Pregnancy in Multiple Sclerosis (PRIMS) study has provided the best large-scale, prospective published data on this issue. The original PRIMS study involved 254 women (246 with relapsing MS and 269 pregnancies), prospectively followed for at least 12 months after delivery.[39] Prepregnancy annualized relapse rate was

---

Box 2
Pregnancy and immune changes

- Shift from Th1 to Th2 cytokine profile
- Increase in $CD4^+CD25^+$ T-regulatory cells
- Decrease in $CD16^+$ natural killer cells
- Tolerance-promoting signaling molecules and pregnancy-specific serum proteins (sHLA-G, CD 200, Fas-ligand, α-fetoprotein, relaxin, early pregnancy factor, pregnancy-specific glycoproteins, indoleamine 2,3-dioxygenase)
- Increase in placenta-derived hormones: estrogens (estriol, estradiol, progesterone)
- Increase in prolactin
- Increase in calcitriol (hormonal vitamin D) norepinephrine
- Changes in hypothalamic-pituitary-adrenal axis hormones (increased corticotropin, cortisol, corticotropin-releasing hormone)
- Migration of fetal cells, cell-free fetal DNA, into maternal circulation (microchimerism)

0.7, which decreased to 0.5 in the first trimester, 0.6 in the second trimester, and 0.2 (P<.001) in the third trimester. Relapse rate increased to 1.2 (P<.001) during the first 3 months postpartum, then returned to prepregnancy levels. Neither breastfeeding nor epidural anesthesia had any effect. The Expanded Disability Status Scale (DSS) score worsened by 0.7 points during 33 months of follow-up. The subsequent formal 2-year postpartum follow-up found that increased prepregnancy relapse rate, increased relapse rate during pregnancy, and a higher Kurtzke DSS score at pregnancy onset correlated in a univariate analysis with postpartum relapse.[43] Such a relapse occurred in 28% of the cohort. In the multivariate analysis the DSS did not remain predictive, whereas MS disease duration at pregnancy onset emerged as a predictive factor (longer duration was at higher risk). Only 72% of the women who relapsed could be correctly identified prospectively, so there was not truly a predictive profile. However, this study helped to generate the POPART'MUS trial, which is looking at progestin (nomegestrol acetate, 10 mg by mouth) plus transdermal endometrial protective doses of estradiol (75 μg weekly) in the postpartum period.[44] The goal is to use sex hormones to suppress postpartum relapses. This ongoing study is due to be completed in 2012. A recent study looked at MRI in 19 MS women, during their third trimester and at 4 to 12 weeks postpartum.[45] Eleven patients (58%) had new or enlarging T2 lesions on their postpartum MRI. An earlier study from this group, involving 28 MS patients, found postpartum clinical or MRI activity in 75%.[46]

In a recent study of 60 radiologically isolated syndrome patients followed for up to 7 years, those who became pregnant (n = 7) were more likely to develop clinical and MRI disease activity,[47] suggesting pregnancy might activate disease in presymptomatic MS. By contrast, an Australian study of clinically isolated syndrome patients, in a comparison with case-matched controls, found that the number of pregnancies was inversely related to the risk of first attack.[48,49] Nulliparous women had a much higher risk for presenting with a clinical attack.

DELIVERY ISSUES

Early delivery (preterm birth) does not increase risk for MS.[50] Birth weight does not affect MS risk.[51] MS does not dictate whether vaginal delivery or cesarean section is preferred. This decision is typically made based on obstetric factors. The one exception would be rare patients with significant baseline neurologic disability whereby they might not be able to push during labor. Again, most pregnant MS patients are relapsing and not disabled. With regard to anesthesia, according to the National MS Society all forms of anesthesia are considered safe for pregnant women. In the PRIMS study no impact of epidural anesthesia was observed. There are anecdotal cases of issues after spinal anesthesia in MS.[52–54] However, there are no convincing data to argue for prohibition of spinal anesthesia.[55]

POSTPARTUM ISSUES

After delivery, about 30% of relapsing MS women have a postpartum relapse.[39] There are several options enabling one to deal with this high-risk period (**Box 3**). In general, breastfeeding is a contraindication to using MS-specific therapy. However, intravenous immunoglobulins (IVIG) have been given in a series of relatively small-scale studies.[15,56–61] IVIG was even pulsed during pregnancy, with reported success.[56] In the recently completed GAMPP study, 173 MS women were randomized to receive either 10-g or 60-g loads of IVIG after delivery, then a monthly pulse of 10 g times 5.[58] Both arms showed similar results, with a return to the prepregnancy relapse by 3 months.

Box 3
Postpartum therapy options during the high-risk period

- Choice is made to breastfeed
  - This is typically associated with withholding of specific MS therapy; however, if treatment is needed one may opt for pulse IVIG for 3 to 6 months, or pulse steroids for 3 to 6 months (delay breastfeeding for 4–6 hours after steroids)
- Choice is made to not breastfeed
  - This is typically associated with resumption or initiation of MS therapy; if there is great concern for disease activity, one may consider combination therapy (pulse IVIG or steroids for 3 to 6 months, with MS therapy)

Pulse intravenous methylprednisolone has also been tried postpartum, with possible benefit.[62] Sex hormones are currently under study in the POPART'MUS trial; these patients are not allowed to breastfeed.[44]

COUNSELING

MS patients should be counseled that MS will not affect their ability to conceive and bear a child. The disease process and their prognosis are not worsened by pregnancy. MS is not an inherited disease; there is no gene that passes on MS. The risk of MS with a first-degree relative with the disease becomes a little higher, 2% to 4% versus 0.2%.[14] There is likely an equal risk of maternal and paternal transmission, although reports have been conflicting.[58,63,64] Epidural anesthesia is safe, and in fact no anesthetic technique is contraindicated. Breastfeeding is safe, and may convey some benefit to controlling disease activity.

MANAGEMENT OF RELAPSES DURING PREGNANCY

It is unusual for a patient to relapse while pregnant, but it can occur and marks them as having an increased risk for a postpartum relapse. Glucocorticoids can be used during pregnancy to treat relapses, typically 1 g of methylprednisolone for 3 to 7 days depending on relapse severity, without oral taper. It is preferred not to use glucocorticoids (if possible) during the first trimester, when organogenesis occurs. Intravenous gammaglobulin is considered safe to use during pregnancy.

PREGNANCY AND THERAPY

None of the MS disease-modifying therapies (DMTs) approved by the Food and Drug Administration (FDA) carries a category-A rating for use in pregnancy (**Table 1**). None of the proposed future agents carries this favorable rating (**Table 2**). Current guidelines from the FDA, and the National MS Society, state that the DMTs should not be used in patients who are trying to become pregnant, who are pregnant, or who are breastfeeding. This advice has been focused on women, with very little attention paid to men.[65] There are no convincing data that the MS DMTs are teratogenic. A study from Argentina reported a higher than expected rate of birth defects with exposure to interferon-β, but numbers were small: 35 women and 42 pregnancies.[66] The interferon-βs are abortofacients in certain animal models, at doses higher than are used in MS. Early, limited small-scale studies suggested that rates of spontaneous abortion and/or smaller birth weight might be higher with interferon-β.[67–70] A later study of 425 exposures showed no increase in abortion rate or congenital anomalies.[71] Glatiramer

Table 1 Pregnancy rating of MS therapies	
FDA-Approved Drug	**Pregnancy Category**
Interferon-β	C
Glatiramer acetate	B
Fingolimod	C
Natalizumab	C
Mitoxantrone	D

acetate has the best pregnancy rating, with no problems reported.[72–74] Overall, no significant issues have been identified with either the interferon-βs or glatiramer acetate.[75–79] Limited data on natalizumab and fingolimod have also not identified a problem. Fingolimod has been associated with developmental toxicity in rats and rabbits, and it is recommended that patients be weaned off fingolimod 2 months before trying to become pregnant. Natalizumab has been associated with miscarriages in guinea pigs and monkeys, and low counts of red blood cells and platelets in newborn monkeys. The limited available publications have not identified any issues with pregnancy in natalizumab-exposed patients.[80–82]

At present most practitioners recommend at least 1 month off therapy before becoming pregnant. Most physicians do not treat pregnant women. Some will, however, particularly with glatiramer acetate.

BREASTFEEDING

Because there are no definitive data on whether the DMTs enter breast milk, breast-feeding is considered a contraindication to treatment by the FDA and National MS Society guidelines.

Exclusive breastfeeding produces prolonged lactational amenorrhea and ovarian suppression.[79] No study has reported a negative effect of breastfeeding on MS. A recent study claimed that exclusive breastfeeding significantly reduced the risk of postpartum relapse,[83] and suggested that anovulation might be protective, although this was a very small nonrandomized study of 32 MS women and 29 controls. A later study from this group reported lower vitamin D levels in the women who exclusively breastfed.[84] In the much larger PRIMS study, breastfeeding was ultimately considered to have no effect on postpartum relapses or disability.[43] It was noted that women who breastfed appeared to do better, but were preselected for milder disease. In a later report from the MS Society Group of the Italian Neurological Society, involving 302 full-term deliveries in 298 MS women, breastfeeding had no impact on relapse

Table 2 Pregnancy rating: future therapies	
Drug	**Pregnancy Category**
Alemtuzumab	C
Anti-CD20 monoclonals	C
BG12	?B/C
Daclizumab	C
Teriflunomide	?C/X

rate.[85] Postpartum relapses were predicted by relapses in the year before pregnancy as well as during pregnancy.

CURRENT RECOMMENDATIONS

Current recommendations should make clear that MS is not a contraindication to pregnancy and that a normal pregnancy and delivery should be expected. Most patients who are pregnant, actively trying to become pregnant, or who are breastfeeding will not be on a DMT, based on current consensus guidelines. Accidental pregnancy should result in discontinuation of therapy. That being said, a patient and physician, if risks/guidelines are clearly understood, might elect to continue therapy; this is most common with glatiramer acetate. There is no clearly defined time to be off treatment before attempting to become pregnant. This time could be immediate with the interferon-βs and glatiramer acetate, or up to 2 months with fingolimod.

During pregnancy, both glucocorticoids and IVIG can be used if needed. Postpartum, about 30% of MS women are at risk of relapse. Risk factors are higher attack rate before pregnancy and attack during pregnancy. Options are resumption of DMT and electing not to breastfeed, or exclusive breastfeeding and delayed resumption of DMT. Pulse IVIG can be offered to either group, as monotherapy or combination therapy. The GAMPP study used either a 10-g or 60-g load, followed by monthly 10-g IVIG infusions over the next 5 months[58]; this was a monotherapy study.

High-risk patients should probably be recommended to receive DMT immediately, and forgo breastfeeding.

FUTURE

It would be very helpful to categorize whether the various DMTs should truly not be used during pregnancy and breastfeeding. It would be instructive to determine the major factors in the last trimester that lead to suppression of MS disease activity. A recent preliminary study evaluated MS pregnancy-related gene-expression pattern changes, and identified 8 transcripts involved in inflammatory processes.[86] It would be invaluable to accurately determine the women at risk for postpartum disease activity. The more one understands how pregnancy and the rapid postpartum changes affect MS, the more insight one may gain into disease pathogenesis and optimal management, including development of new treatment strategies.

SUMMARY

Pregnancy is the best studied hormonal state in MS, and there is sufficient information to provide reliable counseling to patients. Understanding why pregnancy affects MS may lead to new disease insights and therapeutic approaches.

REFERENCES

1. Chao MJ, Ramagopalan SV, Herrera BM, et al. MHC transmission. Insights into gender bias in MS susceptibility. Neurology 2011;76:242–6.
2. Gardener H, Munger KL, Chitnis T, et al. Prenatal and perinatal factors and risk of multiple sclerosis. Epidemiology 2009;20:611–8.
3. Hedstrom AK, Akerstedt T, Hillert J, et al. Shift work at young age is associated with increased risk for multiple sclerosis. Ann Neurol 2011;70(5):733–41.
4. Staples J, Ponsonby AL, Lim L. Low maternal exposure to ultraviolet radiation in pregnancy, month of birth, and risk of multiple sclerosis in offspring: longitudinal analysis. BMJ 2010;340:c1640.

5. Montgomery SM, Bahmanyar S, Hillert J, et al. Maternal smoking during pregnancy and multiple sclerosis amongst offspring. Eur J Neurol 2008;15:1395–9.
6. Mirzaei F, Michels KB, Munger K, et al. Gestational vitamin D and the risk of multiple sclerosis in offspring. Ann Neurol 2011;70:30–40.
7. Moll NM, Rietsch AM, Thomas S, et al. Multiple sclerosis normal-appearing white matter: pathology-imaging correlations. Ann Neurol 2011;70:764–73.
8. Jobin C, Larochelle C, Parpal H, et al. Gender issues in multiple sclerosis: an update. Womens Health (Lond Engl) 2010;6:797–820.
9. Coyle PK, Curkendall S, Johnson BH, et al. Prevalence of Pregnancy in Multiple Sclerosis [abstract]. Neurology 2011;76(Suppl 4):A611.
10. Hellwig K, Brune N, Haghikia A, et al. Reproductive counseling, treatment and course of pregnancy in 73 German MS patients. Acta Neurol Scand 2008;118: 24–8.
11. Laplaud DA, Leray E, Barriere P, et al. Increase in multiple sclerosis relapse rate following in vitro fertilization. Neurology 2006;66:1280–1.
12. Hellwig K, Beste C, Brune N, et al. Increased MS relapse rate during assisted reproduction technique. J Neurol 2008;255:592–3.
13. Hellwig K, Schimrigk S, Beste C, et al. Increase in relapse rate during assisted reproduction technique in patients with multiple sclerosis. Eur Neurol 2009;61:65–8.
14. Lee M, O'Brien P. Multiple sclerosis and pregnancy. J Neurol Neurosurg Psychiatry 2006;79:1308–11.
15. Vukusic S, Confavreux C. Pregnancy and multiple sclerosis: the children of PRIMS. Clin Neurol Neurosurg 2006;108:266–70.
16. Runmarker B, Andersen O. Pregnancy is associated with a lower risk of onset and a better prognosis in multiple sclerosis. Brain 1995;118:253–61.
17. D'hooghe MB, Nagels G, Uitdehaag BM. Long-term effects of childbirth in MS. J Neurol Neurosurg Psychiatry 2010;81:38–41.
18. Verdru P, Theys P, D'hooghe MB, et al. Pregnancy and multiple sclerosis: the influence on long-term disability. Clin Neurol Neurosurg 1994;96:38–41.
19. D'hooghe MB, Haentjens P, Nagels G, et al. Menarche, oral contraceptives, pregnancy and progression of disability in relapsing onset and progressive onset multiple sclerosis. J Neurol 2012;259(5):855–61.
20. Koch M, Uyttenboogaart M, Heersema D, et al. Parity and secondary progression in multiple sclerosis. J Neurol Neurosurg Psychiatry 2009;80:676–8.
21. Finkelsztejn A, Brooks JBB, Paschoal FM Jr, et al. What can we really tell women with multiple sclerosis regarding their pregnancy? A systematic review and meta-analysis of the literature. BJOG 2011;118:790–7.
22. Tsui A, Lee MA. Multiple sclerosis and pregnancy. Curr Opin Obstet Gynecol 2011;23:435–9.
23. Chen YH, Lin HL, Lin HC. Does multiple sclerosis increase risk of adverse pregnancy outcomes? A population-based study. Mult Scler 2009;15:606–12.
24. Dahl J, Myhr KM, Daltveit AK, et al. Pregnancy, delivery and birth outcome in different stages of maternal multiple sclerosis. J Neurol 2008;255:623–7.
25. Jalkanen A, Alanen A, Airas L, et al. Pregnancy outcome in women with multiple sclerosis: results from a prospective nationwide study in Finland. Mult Scler 2010; 16:950–5.
26. van der Kop ML, Pearce MS, Dahlgren L, et al. Neonatal and delivery outcomes in women with multiple sclerosis. Ann Neurol 2011;70:41–50.
27. Airas L, Nikula T, Huang YH, et al. Postpartum activation of multiple sclerosis is associated with down-regulation of tolerogenic HLA-G. J Neuroimmunol 2007; 187:205–11.

28. Bloch EM, Reed WF, Lee TH, et al. Male microchimerism in peripheral blood leukocytes from women with multiple sclerosis. Chimerism 2011;2:6–10.
29. Borchers AT, Naguwa SM, Keen CL, et al. The implications of autoimmunity and pregnancy. J Autoimmun 2010;34:287–99.
30. Kumpel BM, Manoussaka MS. Placental immunology and maternal alloimmune responses. Vox Sang 2012;102:2–12.
31. Langer-Gould A, Gupta R, Huang S, et al. Interferon-γ-producing T cells, pregnancy, and postpartum relapse of multiple sclerosis. Arch Neurol 2010;67: 51–7.
32. Lashley L, van der Hoorn ML, van der Mast BJ, et al. Changes in cytokine production and composition of peripheral blood leukocytes during pregnancy are not associated with a difference in the proliferative immune response to the fetus. Hum Immunol 2011;72:805–11.
33. Neuteboom RF, Verbraak E, Wierenga-Wolf AF, et al. Pregnancy-induced fluctuations in functional T-cell subsets in multiple sclerosis patients. Mult Scler 2010;16: 1073–8.
34. Nicot AB. Gender and sex hormones in multiple sclerosis pathology and therapy. Front Biosci 2009;14:4477–515.
35. Nikbin B, Bonab MM, Talebian F. Microchimerism and stem cell transplantation in multiple sclerosis. Int Rev Neurobiol 2007;79:173–202.
36. Nussinovitch U, Shoenfeld Y. The role of gender and organ specific autoimmunity. Autoimmun Rev 2012;11(6-7):A377–85.
37. Saraste M, Vaisanen S, Alanen A, et al. Clinical and immunologic evaluation of women with multiple sclerosis during and after pregnancy. Gend Med 2007;4: 45–55.
38. Willer CJ, Herrera BM, Morrison KM, et al. Association between microchimerism and multiple sclerosis in Canadian twins. J Neuroimmunol 2006;179:145–51.
39. Confavreux C, Hutchinson M, Hours MM, et al. Rate of pregnancy-related relapse in multiple sclerosis. N Engl J Med 1998;339:285–91.
40. Van Walderven MA, Tas MW, Barkhof F, et al. Magnetic resonance evaluation of disease activity during pregnancy in multiple sclerosis. Neurology 1994;44:327–9.
41. Holmqvist P, Hammar M, Landtblom AM, et al. Age at onset of multiple sclerosis is correlated to use of combined oral contraceptives and childbirth before diagnosis. Fertil Steril 2010;94:2835–7.
42. Nielsen NM, Jorgensen KT, Stenager E, et al. Reproductive history and risk of multiple sclerosis. Epidemiology 2011;22:546–52.
43. Vukusic S, Hutchinson M, Hours M, et al. Pregnancy and multiple sclerosis (the PRIMS study): clinical predictors of postpartum relapse. Brain 2004;127: 1353–60.
44. Vukusic S, Ionescu I, El-Etr M, et al. The prevention of postpartum relapses with Progestin and Estradiol in multiple sclerosis (POPART'MUS) trial: rationale, objectives and state of advancement. J Neurol Sci 2009;286:114–8.
45. Paavilainen T, Kurki T, Färkkilä M, et al. Lower brain diffusivity in postpartum period compared to late pregnancy: results from a prospective imaging study of multiple sclerosis patients. Neuroradiology 2011. [Epub ahead of print].
46. Paavilainen T, Kurki T, Parkkola R, et al. Magnetic resonance imaging of the brain used to detect early postpartum activation of multiple sclerosis. Eur J Neurol 2007;14:1216–21.
47. Lebrun C, Le Page E, Kantarci O, et al. Impact of pregnancy on conversion to clinically isolated syndrome in a radiologically isolated syndrome cohort. Mult Scler 2012. [Epub ahead of print].

48. Ponsonby AL, Lucas RM, van der Mei IA, et al. Offspring number, pregnancy, and risk of a first clinical demyelinating event: the autoimmune study. Neurology 2012; 78:967–74.
49. Daumer M, Weinshenker BG, Voskuhl R. Pregnancy: a "modifiable" risk factor in MS? Neurology 2012;78:846–8.
50. Ramagopalan SV, Valdar W, Dyment DA, et al. No effect of preterm birth on the risk of multiple sclerosis: a population based study. BMC Neurol 2008;8:30.
51. Ramagopalan SV, Herrera BM, Valdar W, et al. No effect of birth weight on the risk of multiple sclerosis. A population-based study. Neuroepidemiology 2008;31: 181–4.
52. Bamford C, Sibley W, Laguna J. Anesthesia in multiple sclerosis. Can J Neurol Sci 1978;5:41–4.
53. Levesque P, Marsepoil T, Venutolo PH, et al. Multiple sclerosis revealed by spinal anesthesia. Ann Fr Anesth Reanim 1988;7:68–70.
54. Stenuit J, Marchand P. Les sequelles de Rachi-Anaesthesie. Acta Neurol Belg 1968;86:626–35.
55. Perlas A, Chan VW. Neuraxial anesthesia and multiple sclerosis. Can J Anaesth 2005;52:454–8.
56. Achiron A, Kishner I, Dolev M, et al. Effect of intravenous immunoglobulin treatment on pregnancy and postpartum-related relapses in multiple sclerosis. J Neurol 2004;251:1133–7.
57. Achiron A, Rotstein Z, Noy S, et al. Intravenous immunoglobulin treatment in the prevention of childbirth-associated acute exacerbations in multiple sclerosis. J Neurol 1996;243:25–8.
58. Haas J, Hommes OR. A dose comparison study of IVIG in postpartum relapsing-remitting multiple sclerosis. Mult Scler 2007;13:900–8.
59. Confavreux C. Intravenous immunoglobulins, pregnancy and multiple sclerosis. J Neurol 2004;251:1138–9.
60. Durelli L, Isoardo G. High-dose intravenous immunoglobulin treatment of multiple sclerosis. Neurol Sci 2002;23:S39–48.
61. Haas J. High dose IVIG in the postpartum period for prevention of exacerbations in MS. Mult Scler 2000;6:S18–20.
62. De Seze J, Chapelotte M, Delalande S, et al. Intravenous corticosteroids in the postpartum period for reduction of acute exacerbations in multiple sclerosis. Mult Scler 2004;10:596–7.
63. Herrera BM, Ramagopalan SV, Orton S, et al. Parental transmission of MS in a population-based Canadian cohort. Neurology 2007;69:1208–12.
64. Hoppenbrouwers IA, Liu F, Aulchenko YS, et al. Maternal transmission of multiple sclerosis in a Dutch population. Arch Neurol 2008;65:345–8.
65. Hellwig K, Haghikia A, Gold R. Parenthood and immunomodulation in patients with multiple sclerosis. J Neurol 2010;257:580–3.
66. Fernandez Liguori N, Klajn D, Acion L, et al. Epidemiological characteristics of pregnancy, delivery, and birth outcome in women with multiple sclerosis in Argentina (EMEMAR study). Mult Scler 2009;15:555–62.
67. Boskovic R, Wide R, Wolpin J, et al. The reproductive effects of beta interferon therapy in pregnancy. Neurology 2005;65:807–11.
68. Hellwig K, Agne H, Gold R. Interferon beta, birth weight and pregnancy in multiple sclerosis. J Neurol 2009;256:830–1.
69. Patti F, Cavallaro T, Lo Fermo S, et al. Is in utero early-exposure to interferon beta a risk factor for pregnancy outcomes in multiple sclerosis? J Neurol 2008;255: 1250–3.

70. Sandberg-Wollheim M, Frank D, Goodwin TM, et al. Pregnancy outcomes during treatment with interferon beta-1a in patients with multiple sclerosis. Neurology 2005;65:802–6.
71. Sandberg-Wollheim M, Alteri E, Stam Moraga M, et al. Pregnancy outcomes in multiple sclerosis following subcutaneous interferon beta-1a therapy. Mult Scler 2011;17:423–30.
72. Coyle PK, Johnson K, Stark Y, et al. Pregnancy outcomes in patients with multiple sclerosis treated with glatiramer acetate (Copaxone). J Neurol Neurosurg Psychiatry 2003;74:443.
73. Fragoso YD, Finkelsztejn A, Kaimen-Maciel DR, et al. Long-term use of glatiramer acetate by 11 pregnant women with multiple sclerosis: a retrospective, multicentre case series. CNS Drugs 2010;24:969–76.
74. Salminen HJ, Leggett H, Boggild M, et al. Glatiramer acetate exposure in pregnancy: preliminary safety and birth outcomes. J Neurol 2010;257:2020–3.
75. Amato MP, Portaccio E, Ghezzi A, et al. Pregnancy and fetal outcomes after interferon-β exposure in multiple sclerosis. Neurology 2010;75:1794–802.
76. De las Heras V, De Andres C, Tellez N, et al. Pregnancy in multiple sclerosis patients treated with immunomodulators prior to or during part of the pregnancy: a descriptive study in the Spanish population. Mult Scler 2007;13:981–4.
77. Finkelsztejn A, Fragoso YD, Ferreira ML, et al. The Brazilian database on pregnancy in multiple sclerosis. Clin Neurol Neurosurg 2011;113:277–80.
78. Lu E, Dahlgren L, Sadovnick AD, et al. Perinatal outcomes in women with multiple sclerosis exposed to disease-modifying drugs. Mult Scler 2012;18(4):460–7.
79. Weber-Schoendorfer C, Schaefer C. Multiple sclerosis, immunomodulators, and pregnancy outcome: a prospective observational study. Mult Scler 2009;15:1037–42.
80. Bayas A, Penzien J, Hellwig K. Accidental natalizumab administration to the third trimester of pregnancy in an adolescent patient with multiple sclerosis. Acta Neurol Scand 2011;124:290–2.
81. Hellwig K, Haghikia A, Gold R. Pregnancy and natalizumab: results of an observational study in 35 accidental pregnancies during natalizumab treatment. Mult Scler 2011;17:958–63.
82. Hoevenaren IA, de Vries LC, Rijnders RJP, et al. Delivery of healthy babies after natalizumab use for multiple sclerosis: a report of two cases. Acta Neurol Scand 2011;123:430–3.
83. Langer-Gould A, Huang SM, Gupta R, et al. Exclusive breastfeeding and the risk of postpartum relapses in women with multiple sclerosis. Arch Neurol 2009;66:958–63.
84. Langer-Gould A, Huang SM, Van Den Eeden SK, et al. Vitamin D, pregnancy, breastfeeding, and postpartum multiple sclerosis relapses. Arch Neurol 2011;68:310–3.
85. Portaccio E, Ghezzi A, Hakiki B, et al. Breastfeeding is not related to postpartum relapses in multiple sclerosis. Neurology 2011;77:145–50.
86. Gilli F, Lindberg RL, Valentino P, et al. Learning from nature: pregnancy changes the expression of inflammation-related genes in patients with multiple sclerosis. PLoS One 2010;5:e8962.

Neuromuscular Disorders in Pregnancy

Amanda C. Guidon, MD[a], E. Wayne Massey, MD[b],*

KEYWORDS

- Neuromuscular diseases • Pregnancy • Neuropathy • Myopathy
- Muscular dystrophy • Myasthenia gravis

KEY POINTS

- Women can develop new neuromuscular disease during pregnancy or in the postpartum period. Pregnancy occurring in patients with neuromuscular disease should be considered in their evaluation, treatment, and prognosis.
- Neurologists can have a critical function in discussing selected pregnancies and facilitating appropriate genetic counseling and prenatal and postnatal care in women with known neuromuscular disease.
- Neurologic treatment choices in women of childbearing potential should include consideration of future pregnancy and the potential effects of therapy on the fetus.
- An individualized plan for pregnancy based on available disease-specific data with early interdisciplinary collaboration is recommended.

INTRODUCTION

Women may develop symptoms of acquired or manifest inherited neuromuscular disorders during pregnancy. For women with preexisting disease, many challenging questions arise for both the patient and the treating physicians surrounding pregnancy and delivery: Will the course of maternal disease change? Will treatment need to be adjusted, and, if so, how? What are the potential effects of therapy on the fetus? Will there be complications during labor and delivery? Are there additional implications for the fetus? The existing literature on the topic consists of isolated case reports and retrospective reviews. Most individual neurologists, including neuromuscular specialists, high-risk obstetricians, and anesthesiologists, have limited personal experience with pregnancy in any particular disorder. The most recent literature on neuromuscular disorders in pregnancy (**Box 1**) is reviewed.

The authors have nothing to disclose.
[a] Division of Neurology, Department of Medicine, Duke University Medical Center, DUMC 3403, Durham, NC 27710, USA; [b] Division of Neurology, Department of Medicine, Duke University Medical Center, DUMC 3909, Durham, NC 27710, USA
* Corresponding author.
E-mail address: masse010@mc.duke.edu

Box 1
Disorders reviewed in pregnancy

I. Root, plexus, peripheral nerve:

Median neuropathy at the wrist (carpal tunnel syndrome [CTS])

Lateral femoral cutaneous neuropathy (meralgia paresthetica)

Lumbar radiculopathy and plexopathy

Sciatic and common fibular (peroneal) neuropathy

Femoral neuropathy

Obturator neuropathy

Idiopathic facial nerve palsy (Bell's palsy)

Radial neuropathy

Intercostal neuralgia

II. Acquired disorders of peripheral nerves

Acute inflammatory demyelinating polyradiculoneuropathy (AIDP)

Chronic inflammatory demyelinating polyradiculoneuropathy (CIDP)

Multifocal motor neuropathy (MMN)

III. Acquired muscle disease

Polymyositis

Dermatomyositis

IV. Disorders of the neuromuscular junction

Myasthenia gravis

V. Inherited Neuropathies

Charcot-Marie-Tooth (CMT) disease

Hereditary neuropathy with liability to pressure palsies (HNPP)

Hereditary brachial plexus neuropathy (HBPN)

VI. Inherited muscle disorders

Facioscapulohumeral muscular dystrophy (FSHD)

Limb-girdle muscular dystrophies

Myotonic dystrophies

Nondystrophic myotonias and periodic paralysis

Congenital nemaline rod myopathy

Metabolic myopathy

Mitochondrial myopathy

VII. Motor neuron disease

Spinal muscular atrophies (SMA)

Amyotrophic lateral sclerosis (ALS)

ACQUIRED ROOT, PLEXUS, AND PERIPHERAL NERVE LESIONS
Median Neuropathy at the Wrist (CTS)

Median neuropathy at the wrist, CTS, is the most frequently occurring compression neuropathy in pregnancy. In a systematic review, the incidence of pregnancy-related CTS (PRCTS) varied greatly in published studies from approximately 1% to 60%. When limited to prospective studies describing only electrodiagnostically confirmed CTS, the incidence in pregnancy was approximately 17%.[1] Symptoms of CTS include pain and paresthesias mainly in the hand and fingers but may include the arm and shoulder. Patients describe hand weakness, clumsiness, and stiffness. In severe cases, atrophy and weakness of the abductor pollicis brevis muscle may develop.[2]

The relationship between CTS and pregnancy is poorly understood. The median nerve crosses from the forearm to the hand through the carpal tunnel. CTS is caused by reduced space within the carpal tunnel or increased susceptibility of the nerve to pressure.[2] It can develop in endocrine or hematologic disorders.[2] Most women who develop PRCTS have the onset of symptoms in their third trimester.[3] Edema in the tissues of the carpal tunnel caused by fluid retention in pregnancy has been hypothesized to induce mechanical compression of the median nerve.[4] An association between gestational diabetes and PRCTS has not been reported.[5] CTS may also develop postpartum while breastfeeding. CTS during lactation does not seem to be associated with edema and may be more common in older, primiparous women.[6]

PRCTS has different characteristics than idiopathic CTS. An Italian cohort of 45 women with PRCTS was compared in their third trimester with age-matched controls with CTS. The pregnant women were more likely to have a shorter duration of symptoms, more frequent bilateral symptoms, more white-collar occupations, and lower clinical and electrophysiologic severity stages than the control group. At 3-year follow-up, a smaller percentage of women in the pregnancy cohort had undergone surgery. Among patients without surgery, 50% of patients in the pregnancy group had symptoms at 3 years compared with 83% of the control group.[3] Clinical improvement may not correlate with electrodiagnostic improvement postpartum.[7] Furthermore, pregnant women without symptoms of CTS may have electrodiagnostic evidence for CTS.[8]

The natural history of PRCTS varies after delivery. Symptoms resolve spontaneously in half of patients after 1 year and in two-thirds by 3 years.[1] Patients with symptom onset earlier in pregnancy and a larger pregnancy-associated weight gain are more likely to have persistent symptoms.[5,7] Given the high rate of spontaneous resolution, many propose that nonoperative treatment should be first-line therapy. Surgery can be considered if conservative measures fail or in severe acute cases with debilitating functional impairment.[1] No randomized data exist comparing the effects of different nonoperative therapies (eg, analgesics, low-salt diet, rest, splinting, local steroid and/or lidocaine injections). Delivery is considered definitive therapy. A higher number of lifetime pregnancies may be a risk factor for idiopathic CTS in postmenopausal women.[9]

Lateral Femoral Cutaneous Neuropathy (Meralgia Paresthetica)

Meralgia paresthetica is a sensory mononeuropathy that occurs from damage to the lateral cutaneous nerve of the thigh (LCNT) (also called the lateral femoral cutaneous nerve). Lesions can occur anywhere along the nerve's highly variable course. Locations of trauma include the psoas muscle, iliacus compartment in the pelvis, inguinal ligament, or the thigh. In many cases, no cause is identified. Symptoms include pain, paresthesias, and numbness in the anterolateral thigh. Physical examination reveals sensory loss over the distribution of the LCNT without motor or reflex changes.

Meralgia paresthetica can occur before or after delivery and can be unilateral or bilateral. Standing, walking, and either flexing or extending the hip can worsen symptoms.[2]

During pregnancy and delivery, the LCNT can be compressed or stretched by several proposed mechanisms. The protuberant abdomen or increased lumbar lordosis may alter the angle between the nerve and the inguinal ligament, causing compression or stretch injury. During labor, compression may occur by the inguinal ligament during maternal pushing with the thighs flexed, increased abdominal pressure and abdominal wall tension during the second stage of labor, or by the elastic belts worn on the abdomen to hold monitors in place. Cutting or retraction during cesarean section may also injure the nerve.[10,11] The nerve is unlikely to be damaged by regional anesthesia because it originates from the L2 to L3 nerve roots at least several centimeters lateral to the transverse process. The presence of meralgia paresthetica should not preclude the use of epidural or spinal anesthesia.

Management of meralgia paresthetica in pregnancy (after it is often mistaken for L2 to L3 disorders with onset) is generally conservative and most cases resolve spontaneously on follow-up several months after delivery. Treatment focuses on avoiding aggravating positions, tight-fitting clothing, and excessive weight gain. Nonsteroidal antiinflammatory drugs, transcutaneous electrical nerve stimulation (TENS), and topical anesthesia with Lidoderm patches (US Food and Drug Administration [FDA] category B) can be used (**Table 1**).[12,13] Anesthetic/steroid injections have been reported. Treatments including tricyclic antidepressants and antiepileptics like gabapentin, pregabalin, and carbamezapine are all category C or D in pregnancy.[11]

Postpartum Foot Drop Caused by Focal Peripheral Nerve and Root Lesions

Nerve injury at the level of the lumbar root, plexus, sciatic nerve, or common fibular (peroneal) nerve can cause foot drop. Physical examination and electrodiagnostic studies help localize the site of the lesion. In general, frequent changes of lower extremity position, avoidance of prolonged thigh flexion or extreme thigh abduction

Table 1 FDA drug classification in pregnancy	
FDA Category	**Summary**
A	Adequate and well-controlled studies in pregnant women have failed to show a risk to the fetus Drug should be used in pregnancy only if needed
B	Animal studies show no risk to the fetus and there are no adequate and well-controlled studies in humans, or fetal risk shown in some animal studies but not confirmed in humans Drug should be used in pregnancy only if needed
C	Animal studies show an adverse effect on the fetus No adequate and well-controlled studies in humans Benefits in pregnant women may be acceptable despite potential risks
D	Studies show evidence of human fetal risk Benefits in pregnant women may be acceptable despite potential risks
X	Studies show evidence of human fetal risk Risk in pregnant women outweighs potential benefit

From US Food and Drug Administration. Department of Health and Human Services. Subchapter C–Drugs: General. Code of Federal Regulations [Online]. Title 21, vol. 4. Revised as of April 1, 2011. Available at: http://www.accessdata.fda.gov/scripts/cdrh/cfdocs/cfCFR/CFRSearch.cfm?CFRPart=201&showFR=1. Accessed May 22, 2012.

and external rotation, and shortened active labor time can be implemented to prevent nerve injury during labor. Epidural anesthesia is associated with a longer second stage of labor. Because of sensory blockade, parturients may not sense pressure on their limbs and change positions frequently enough on their own to prevent injury.[10]

Low back pain from musculoskeletal causes is reported in approximately 50% of pregnancies. However, low back pain caused by a hernatiated disc occurs in only 1 in 10,000 pregnancies. Pregnancy itself does not increase the risk of disc herniation.[14,15] Radiculopathy can occur because of disc disease, tumor, trauma, inflammation, and infection.[10] Radiating back pain with abnormal lower limb sensation, strength, or deep tendon reflexes is concerning for a lumbosacral radiculopathy and should prompt evaluation with noncontrasted magnetic resonance imaging (MRI) of the lumbar spine and electrodiagnostic studies. Gadolinium contrast agents cross the placenta and are excreted by the fetal kidneys into the amniotic fluid. They are classified as pregnancy category C and should be used only if the potential benefit outweighs the risk.[16] Most common causes of low back pain and radiculopathy may be evaluated without gadolinium contrast agents. However, gadolinium may be considered if infection, inflammation, or malignancy are of concern.[17] Cauda equina syndrome from lumbar disc herniation presents with radiating back pain, sphincter disturbance, saddle anesthesia, weakness, and loss of Achilles reflexes. Although rare in pregnancy and the postpartum period, it is a neurosurgical emergency.[15] There is a single report of a known lumbar disc herniation that progressed to cauda equina syndrome after cesarean section.[18] Preexisting low back pain and disc herniation may worsen during pregnancy. Surgery can be performed safely in pregnant patients with progressive neurologic deficits caused by disc herniation.[15] Back pain without neurologic deficits can often be managed conservatively during pregnancy.

The optimal method of delivery and anesthesia in pregnant women with known lumbar disc herniation is debated. Most investigators advocate cesarean section to avoid a theoretic worsening of herniation with Valsalva.[18] A low risk of neurologic injury estimated at 0.1% exists with epidural anesthesia. Potential mechanisms of injury include epidural hematoma, drug toxicity, chemical radiculitis, arachnoiditis, and direct needle or injection injury to the nerve root. Women who develop myelopathy or persistent radiculopathy symptoms after epidural anesthesia should undergo urgent MRI of the lumbar spine.[19]

Injuries to the lumbosacral plexus can occur from compression by the fetal head during the second stage of labor or from forceps delivery. Fetal macrosomia, malpresentations, and specific pelvic features are risk factors. Rare injuries to the sciatic nerve have been reported postpartum, although the mechanism of injury is unclear. Common fibular neuropathy in pregnancy is most often caused by external compression. This compression can be caused by inappropriate positioning in leg stirrups, a hyper-flexed knee position with gripping at the fibular head, or by prolonged squatting.[10]

Femoral Neuropathy

The femoral nerve arises from the lumbar plexus and is formed by L2 to L4 nerve roots. It passes between the psoas and iliacus muscles and lateral to the femoral artery under the inguinal ligament. In femoral neuropathies, weakness may be observed involving the quadriceps femoris and iliopsoas, which also receives direct innervation from the plexus. Numbness and paresthesia can be seen in the cutaneous distribution of the femoral and saphenous nerve over the distal anteromedial thigh and medial aspect of the lower leg. Associated pain is variable. In severe lesions, weakness and atrophy of the quadriceps muscle and absence of the patellar reflex are present.

Involvement of both hip flexion and adduction suggests a root or lumbosacral plexus disorder.[2]

Femoral neuropathy in pregnancy is rare and incidence has likely decreased over time because of changes in obstetric management. In one retrospective review, femoral neuropathy occurred in approximately 0.3% of 6057 live births. Primiparous women with a prolonged second stage of labor were more likely to develop femoral neuropathy.[10] The lithotomy position may cause compression of the femoral nerve at the inguinal ligament and stretch the nerve through excessive hip abduction and external rotation.[20] Treatment is supportive and the average time to recovery is approximately 2 to 6 months.[10]

Obturator Neuropathy

The obturator nerve is formed within the psoas muscle from the anterior divisions of the ventral rami of the L2 to L4 roots. It descends through the pelvis and exits through the obturator foramen, supplying motor innervation to hip adductor muscles and sensory fibers to a small area on the upper medial thigh.[2] Obturator neuropathies have rarely been reported in the postpartum period; weakness of hip adduction is more likely to be caused by a lumbar (L3/L4) radiculopathy or plexopathy. The obturator nerve traverses the pelvic brim and can be compressed between the pelvis and fetal head or by forceps. The angle of the nerve as it leaves the obturator foramen changes in the lithotomy position. Hematomas reported from pudendal nerve blocks have been associated with entrapment neuropathies of the obturator nerve. Duration of symptoms in 3 patients studied with obturator neuropathies postpartum was similar to other lower extremity neuropathies associated with delivery.[10]

Idiopathic Facial Nerve Palsy (Bell's Palsy)

During pregnancy and the postpartum period, Bell's palsy occurs in 38 to 45.1 per 100,000 births, 3.3 times the rate per year in nonpregnant women of childbearing age.[21] Most cases occur in the third trimester or early postpartum period.[22,23]

Although the pathophysiology of Bell's palsy in pregnancy is poorly understood, viral infection, vascular ischemia, autoimmune inflammatory disorders, and hereditary factors have been proposed mechanisms in the general population. Some speculate that relative immunosuppression in pregnancy may lower the threshold for reactivation of herpes simplex or zoster viruses from the geniculate ganglia, resulting in Bell's palsy.[24] The correlation between the timing of maximum extracellular fluid volume and the peak incidence in pregnancy has led others to hypothesize a mechanical compressive mechanism. Changing levels of estrogen and progesterone, increased cortisol levels, hypertension, preeclampsia, and hypercoagulable states in the third trimester have also been invoked.[22] Retrospective studies have reported a significant and independent association with chronic or gestational hypertension, preeclampsia, and obesity. Two studies have shown higher rates of cesarean section. However, there are conflicting data about the association with adverse perinatal outcomes including low Apgar scores, perinatal mortality, or fetal malformation.[23,25]

Although most patients regain near normal function, retrospective data suggest that pregnant women are more likely to progress toward complete facial paralysis. In addition, those with complete paralysis are more likely to have an unsatisfactory recovery compared with the nonpregnant population. Whether this difference is caused by the disease process or differences in treatment patterns during pregnancy is not known.[22] Pregnant and breastfeeding women have generally been excluded from trials exploring therapy with corticosteroids and antiviral agents, although corticosteroids are generally safe in pregnancy.

Radial Neuropathy

Inappropriate placement of the arms while using the birthing bar during labor can lead to compression of the radial nerve at the spiral groove. One patient was reported to have bilateral wrist drop and finger extension weakness 8 hours postpartum after using the birthing bar for several hours during her second stage of labor. Electro-diagnostic studies confirmed bilateral radial neuropathies. On follow-up at 1 year, she had regained 80% of her strength. Special caution is encouraged in patients who receive epidurals because they might place more weight on their arms while using a birthing bar.[26]

Intercostal Neuralgia

Intercostal neuralgia (also called thoraconeuralgia gravidarum) is a rare disorder in pregnancy, characterized by sensory changes and significant pain in the distribution of a thoracic root or intercostal nerve. All reported patients were affected in the lower thoracic region. Pain can radiate to the abdomen and may worsen with position or palpation over the paraspinal muscles. Electromyography may exhibit abnormal spontaneous activity in the thoracic paraspinal muscles at the corresponding spinal level, suggesting a radicular syndrome. The cause is unknown. The rapid resolution of symptoms after delivery suggests a physiologic cause rather than a nerve injury that would require remyelination. Symptoms generally remit within hours after delivery. Recurrence of symptoms typically occurs in subsequent pregnancies.[27,28] Treatment with topical lidocaine patches can be considered. One patient was treated successfully with extended epidural local anesthetic until delivery.[29] Neuropathic thoracic pain during pregnancy has various causes including spinal cord lesions, radiculopathy, and irritation of nerve trunks, which must be considered in addition to intra-abdominal disorders in the differential diagnosis for intercostal neuralgia.[27]

ACQUIRED DISORDERS OF PERIPHERAL NERVES
Acute Inflammatory Demyelinating Polyradiculoneuropathy

Acute inflammatory demyelinating polyradiculoneuropathy (AIDP), or Guillain-Barré syndrome (GBS), is an acute neuropathy characterized by progressive weakness, sensory disturbance, and loss of deep tendon reflexes that often follows an ascending pattern. Facial weakness, eye movement abnormalities, autonomic dysfunction, and respiratory compromise may be present.[30] The incidence of GBS is approximately 0.75 to 2 in 100,000 per year, with higher incidence with increasing age. During pregnancy, the age-adjusted incidence is identical to that in the general population. Nearly 90% of these cases occur in the second and third trimesters. GBS occurs nearly 3 times more often in the period 30 days postpartum.[31] Pregnant women may be less likely than the general population to have serologic evidence of associated *Campylobacter jejuni* infection.[32] In the pregnant group, cytomegalovirus (CMV) infection was reported in approximately 10%, which mirrors the general population. Testing for these agents is recommended because their presence is often associated with more severe disease and residual disability and may have significant implications for the developing fetus.[31]

In one review, most patients received treatment with either plasma exchange or intravenous immune globulin (IVIG) with no treatment-related complications reported. Termination of pregnancy did not shorten disease duration or improve maternal outcome. There was no neonatal death and the perinatal survival rate was 96%. Thirty-five percent of patients had preterm delivery, with most caused by labor induced for maternal neurologic decline.[31] Sixty-one percent of patients delivered via cesarean section. However, vaginal deliveries were achieved despite severe weakness and ventilator dependence. Operative delivery should be reserved for obstetric indications. General anesthesia has been used without complication, but may be complicated by autonomic instability. There is 1 report of maternal death from cardiac arrest secondary to hyperkalemia shortly after administration of succinylcholine. Spinal and spinal-epidural anesthesia has been used in this group without complications. One patient had worsening weakness after epidural anesthesia.[33] Prevention of complications from infection and venous thromboembolism is of paramount importance.

Chronic Inflammatory Demyelinating Polyradiculoneuropathy

Chronic inflammatory demyelinating polyradiculoneuropathy (CIDP) is a group of immune-mediated neuropathies with a relapsing or progressive course. They usually present in adults, with a peak incidence between the ages of 40 and 60 years.[30] CIDP in pregnancy is uncommon. In case reports and a small case series of 9 women with CIDP who became pregnant, there was an increased risk of relapse during the third trimester and postpartum periods.[34]

Multifocal Motor Neuropathy

Multifocal motor neuropathy (MMN) is a chronic, immune-mediated neuropathy, characterized by asymmetric, predominantly distal limb weakness and conduction block on motor nerve conduction studies. Anti-GM1 immunoglobulin (Ig) M antibodies are often present.[35] Weakness in existing muscles may worsen and new muscles may become involved during pregnancy. Women generally return to their prepregnancy strength and can be treated with IVIG during pregnancy.[36]

One case of neonatal transmission of an MMN associated with anti-GM1 IgG and IgGλ monoclonal gammopathy has been reported. The infant had decreased fetal movement in utero, distal upper and lower extremity weakness, and hyporeflexia at birth that improved over 1 month. The infant's serum, which normalized after several months, initially showed the same abnormalities. He had persistent distal weakness and atrophy at age 4 years.[37]

ACQUIRED DISORDERS OF MUSCLE
Inflammatory Muscle Disease

The association of idiopathic inflammatory myopathies, dermatomyositis (DM), and polymyositis (PM) with pregnancy is uncommon, likely because of the low percentage of cases (14%) that occur in women of childbearing age. The effect of the disease on fertility is unknown. Exacerbations of previously stable disease in pregnancy are rare and the risk of exacerbations has not been reported. In general, the course and outcome of the pregnancy seems to parallel the activity of maternal disease. Women who are stable on low-dose prednisone at the time of pregnancy generally have uneventful pregnancies and deliveries, and healthy infants. Pregnant women with active disease have an increased risk of obstetric complications, prematurity, and fetal loss.[38,39] In the largest retrospective review published to date, approximately 43% of pregnancies in women with active disease were complicated by fetal death in utero or immediately after delivery, and 33% by intrauterine growth retardation (IUGR)/premature delivery. In contrast, these complications occurred in 13% of women with stable disease.[39]

Treatment during pregnancy generally uses corticosteroids. Flares can often be managed by increasing the dose of prednisone. Chemotherapeutic agents are typically reserved for fulminant or life-threatening disease in pregnancy because of the potential teratogenic effects.[39] IVIG has been used as monotherapy[40] or in combination with high-dose steroids[41] to treat women who presented in the first trimester of pregnancy. Treatment has resulted in remission of maternal disease and the delivery of a healthy infant. The preferred method of delivery has not been studied. DM and PM do not affect smooth muscle and uncomplicated vaginal deliveries have been reported. Some advocate evaluating patients for cesarean section based on the degree of maternal weakness, desire to avoid maternal exertion, and to decrease the possible risk of rhabdomyolysis and myoglobinuria. PM and DM are not transmitted to the fetus. For unknown reasons, asymptomatic newborns may have transiently increased creatine kinase (CK) levels for 2 to 4 months after delivery.[42]

DISORDERS OF THE NEUROMUSCULAR JUNCTION
Myasthenia Gravis

Acquired myasthenia gravis (MG) is an autoimmune disorder in which antibodies at the neuromuscular junction cause impaired neuromuscular transmission and fatigable weakness in skeletal muscle. Disease onset may occur at any age, but female incidence peaks in the third decade. Overall, the disease is more common in women, in a ratio of 3:2. Certain medications, infection, surgery, general anesthesia, emotional stress, menses, pregnancy, and the postpartum state may trigger exacerbations. Most woman of childbearing age with MG have thymomas and acetylcholine receptor (AChR) antibodies.[43,44] MG can first present during pregnancy or the postpartum period. Exacerbations may also occur in patients with preexisting MG. The effect of pregnancy on MG is variable and unpredictable. The effect of one pregnancy on MG does not predict the effect in subsequent pregnancies. Clinical status does not reliably predict the course of MG during pregnancy.[44] In asymptomatic patients not on therapy before pregnancy, approximately 20% have a relapse.[43] In patients on therapy at the time of pregnancy, MG improves in approximately 30% to 40%, remains unchanged 30% to 40%, and worsens in 20% to 30%. The greatest percentage of exacerbations occur in the first trimester, final 4 weeks of gestation, or puerperium.[43,45,46] Infection and shorter history of disease increase the risk of exacerbation in the puerperium.[46] Woman with MG should ideally seek counseling well in advance of becoming pregnant to address the need for thymectomy, reevaluate the use of immunosuppressive therapy, and to maximize clinical improvement. Throughout pregnancy and the postpartum period, an individualized, interdisciplinary approach is needed.

The severity and distribution of weakness should guide therapy decisions for women with MG who are pregnant or planning pregnancy. Initiation of immunosuppressive agents other than prednisone is typically avoided before or during pregnancy. The risk of precipitating exacerbation or crisis by withdrawing immunosuppressive therapy must be weighed against potential harm to the fetus. If thymectomy is indicated, it should be performed before pregnancy or after the postpartum period because of the delayed therapeutic effect and surgical risk. Anticholinesterase medications may be used in pregnancy for symptomatic relief and are pregnancy category C. The dose may need more frequent adjustment because of changes in intestinal absorption and renal clearance. Prednisone and prednisolone are pregnancy category C. A small increase in cleft palate has been reported with use in the first trimester, as well as premature rupture of membrane with high doses. Cyclosporine is also category C and, although its use is generally discouraged in pregnant women with MG, the risk of fetal malformations is low. Concern exists over a possible increased risk of spontaneous abortions, prematurity, and low birth weight. Azathioprine and mycophenolate mofetil are pregnancy category D and methotrexate category X. These medications pose significant risk to the fetus and their use is not recommended in pregnancy.[44]

The risks of IVIG and plasma exchange in pregnancy should be weighed against the potential benefit. Generally, they can be used to manage severe MG symptoms or crisis in pregnancy. IVIG is pregnancy category C and frequently used during pregnancy in many autoimmune conditions. It is generally well tolerated, with few major or minor side effects. The effect on the fetus is unknown. Particular attention should be given in pregnancy to the side effects of hyperviscosity and volume overload. Plasma exchange can be used safely in pregnancy. A left lateral decubitus position and careful monitoring of fluid status protect against hypotension. During the third trimester, fetal monitoring is recommended.[44] The American Academy of Pediatrics considers pyridostigmine, prednisone, and prednisolone compatible with lactation. Azathioprine, cyclosporine, and methotrexate are unsafe during breastfeeding. The safety of mycophenolate mofetil is unknown.[47]

Data regarding the possible increased risk of labor complications are conflicting. MG typically does not affect the first stage of labor, which depends on smooth muscle contraction. The obstetrician should be prepared to assist with vacuum or forceps if fatigue occurs in the second stage of labor, which relies on striated muscle. Cholinesterase inhibitors can help minimize fatigable weakness during the second stage of labor. In one population, total and elective cesarean sections occurred more frequently in woman with MG than in the general population. However, total vacuum or forceps deliveries were no more common.[48] Another study reported no statistically significant difference in the rate of cesarean section or assisted vaginal delivery.[45] Cesarean section is performed only for standard obstetric indications. The mode of delivery does not seem to affect the rate of exacerbation in the puerperium.[46]

Some investigators recommend using regional anesthesia early in labor. Regional anesthesia can be used safely and a low concentration of local anesthetic lessens the risk of motor block. Regional anesthesia is recommended for cesarean section but may exacerbate underlying skeletal muscle weakness. A high level of spinal or epidural anesthesia may impair respiratory function, especially in patients with significant bulbar or respiratory weakness. Individuals with MG have a marked sensitivity to nondepolarizing agents. If their use cannot be avoided in general anesthesia, reduced doses of immediate-acting drugs may be carefully titrated to effect.[49]

Magnesium sulfate should be used with extreme caution for the management of eclampsia. Magnesium blocks calcium entry at the nerve terminal and inhibits ACh release, further disrupting neuromuscular transmission. A case report of magnesium given to a woman with undiagnosed MG for eclampsia resulted in worsening weakness in a dose-dependant fashion. Although serum magnesium levels were slightly more than the upper limit of normal, she developed severe facial and limb weakness that was reversible over the course of 24 hours.[50] If the potential benefit of giving magnesium outweighs the risk, the treating team should be prepared for potential worsening of MG.

No significant differences have been found in MG regarding prematurity, perinatal mortality, birth weight, mean gestational age, or parity.[45,48] Although the total rate of labor complications may be higher in women with MG, premature rupture of the amniotic membranes is the only single complication that occurs more frequently. The overall rate of severe birth defects is not significantly higher. However, infants who have birth defects may be more likely to have skeletal anomalies, possibly caused by placental transfer of anti-AChR antibodies.[48]

Neonatal MG and Arthrogryposis

Transient neonatal MG (TNMG) affects 10% to 15% of infants born to mothers with MG because of transplacental transfer of maternal AChR antibodies to the infant. It is unknown why a small percentage of infants develop symptoms when most have detectable maternal antibodies. Symptoms of TNMG include hypotonia and respiratory, feeding, and swallowing problems. These symptoms typically resolve in an average of 3 weeks (range of 1–7 weeks) and can be treated with supportive care and cholinesterase inhibitors.[51] Symptom severity ranges from mild weakness to respiratory distress requiring ventilatory support. Persistent bulbar and facial weakness and hearing loss following TNMG have been reported. It is hypothesized that this phenotype results from inactivation of the fetal subunit of the acetylcholine receptor during a critical period of fetal muscle development. In these mothers, the fetal/adult AChR ratio was a strong predictor of phenotypic severity in the offspring. Case report data suggest that plasma exchange and possibly prednisone during pregnancy may reduce phenotypic severity in offspring.[52] Before the role of muscle specific kinase (MuSK) antibodies was known in MG, seronegative mothers were reported to have offspring with TNMG. TNMG has since been reported with anti-MuSK antibodies.[53] Rarely, MG is associated with arthrogryposis multiplex congenital (AMC), a disorder characterized by multiple joint contractures and other anomalies, likely from decreased fetal movement in utero. The effect of treating mothers with plasma exchange or immunosuppression during pregnancy on the incidence of neonatal MG is unknown.[54] One child affected with neonatal MG is a strong predictor of subsequent offspring being affected.[52]

Pregnancy in nonparaneoplastic Lambert-Eaton myasthenic syndrome has been reported. One infant had normal intrauterine development and was born without muscle weakness or voltage-gated calcium channel antibodies.[55] Another infant had increased anti-VGCC AB titers and respiratory distress, muscular hypotonia, and sucking and feeding difficulties that lasted for 1 week.[56]

INHERITED DISORDERS OF PERIPHERAL NERVES
Charcot-Marie-Tooth Disease

CMT type 1 (CMT1) is the most common form of hereditary neuropathy. Individuals usually present in the first to third decades with distal lower extremity weakness and hyporeflexia. Although sensory loss may be present on examination, initially, people with CMT1 do not typically complain of numbness or tingling.[30] Data on CMT in pregnancy are from 2 retrospective studies for a total of 153 pregnancies in 70 affected women.[57,58] Most women had CMT1. Pregnancy did not influence symptom severity in patients with adult-onset disease. However, 50% of women with subjective symptoms since youth reported exacerbation of symptoms during pregnancy. Age at delivery, time interval between symptom onset and delivery, and number of prior gestations were no different in the group with exacerbation during pregnancy. Worsening was temporary in approximately 35% and persistent in 65% of patients. Patients who experienced deterioration in their first pregnancy generally had a high risk of deterioration in subsequent pregnancies.[58]

In both studies, total complication rate and perinatal mortality were comparable with a reference population. However, 1 review found a higher occurrence of specific complications including presentation anomalies (eg, breech or abnormal cephalic presentations) and bleeding postpartum. The investigators hypothesized that the CMT genotype in some fetuses may produce decreased movement in utero, although maternal factors cannot be excluded. Postpartum bleeding was possibly related to a CMT-mediated neuropathy of the uterine adrenergic nerves causing uterine atony. Operative delivery occurred twice as frequently and most cesarean sections occurred emergently. Forceps were used 3 times as frequently.[57]

Hereditary Neuropathy with Liability to Pressure Palsies

Hereditary neuropathy with liability to pressure palsies (HNPP) is a generalized demyelinating neuropathy with autosomal dominant inheritance and variable penetrance. Patients experience recurrent, painless focal neuropathies that typically resolve. They often occur at common entrapment sites with minor trauma or compression. Case reports exist of women with HNPP who developed neuropathies from compression during pregnancy and after delivery.[59–61]

Hereditary Brachial Plexus Neuropathy

Hereditary brachial plexus neuropathy (HBPN) is an inherited disorder characterized by periodic attacks of pain, weakness, atrophy, and sensory changes in the upper extremity caused by involvement of the brachial plexus. Although genetically heterogeneous, a mutation in the SEPT9 gene has been reported in several affected families.[62] The cause is thought to be altered immunity and resulting inflammation. Repeated episodes, especially postpartum, a family history, and the presence of mild dysmorphic features help distinguish HBPN from immune brachial plexus neuropathy (Parsonage-Turner syndrome). In one series of 246 patients, 4 of the 10 cases of neuralgic amyotrophy associated with pregnancy were HBPN, whereas the remaining 6 were Parsonage-Turner syndrome.[62] Postpartum attacks in HBPN can occur after both vaginal delivery and cesarean section. Episodes may be treated acutely with intravenous methylprednisolone.[63]

INHERITED DISORDERS OF MUSCLE
Facioscapulohumeral Muscular Dystrophy

Facioscapulohumeral muscular dystrophy (FSHD) is an autosomal dominant disorder with variable penetrance and an incidence of approximately 4 per million. Onset of weakness typically occurs between 3 and 44 years of age in a characteristic pattern involving muscles of facial expression, scapula-stabilizers, biceps brachii, triceps, tibialis anterior, and pelvic muscles.[30] In one retrospective study of 38 women with mild to moderate disability from FSHD, the diagnosis was known at the time of pregnancy in approximately half. Outcomes of the 105 pregnancies in this group were generally good. There were higher rates of cesarean sections and forceps-assisted deliveries compared with the national average, likely because of a compromised second stage of labor when skeletal muscle effort is required. Abdominal and truncal muscle weakness is commonly seen even in mild disease. The incidence of miscarriage, preterm labor, birth defects, and neonatal and perinatal death was equal to the national average. However, the FSHD group had higher rates of low birth weight. Approximately 25% of the pregnancies resulted in exacerbation of muscle weakness and pain that generally did not return to baseline after childbirth. Despite this worsening, nearly all the women surveyed reported that they would choose pregnancy again. Six of the 10 nulliparous women in the cohort reported that they had decided against pregnancy because of their disease.[64] A smaller retrospective study of 11 patients with FSHD reported pregnancy and delivery characteristics equal to the general population. Approximately 25% of this group also reported worsening during pregnancy but had returned to baseline after delivery.[65]

Limb-Girdle Muscular Dystrophies

The limb-girdle muscular dystrophies (LGMD) are a heterogeneous group of myopathies with variable inheritance characterized by progressive weakness in limb-girdle muscles. In one retrospective study of 12 live births to 9 women, there were no miscarriages or preterm births. Five women had obstetric complications resulting in surgical vaginal delivery or cesarean section caused by prolonged labor. All infants were healthy except 1 with a neural tube defect and 1 who died of a respiratory infection at 6 months. More than 50% of women reported weight-related worsening of weakness during pregnancy that generally did not improve. However, all women attributed this worsening to the expected progression of disease. Five women needed assistance from families after delivery to care for their infants. Despite this, they reported a positive attitude toward pregnancy and emphasized the value of family life despite their physical limitations.[65]

Myotonic Dystrophies

Myotonic dystrophy type 1 (DM1) is a multisystem disorder characterized by slowly progressive limb, neck, and facial weakness with myotonia. Inheritance is autosomal dominant, onset of symptoms can occur at any age, and prevalence is 3 to 5 per 100,000. The severity of symptoms directly correlates with the size of the unstable cytosine-thymine-guanine (CTG) trinucleotide repeat in the untranslated 3' region on the myotonin protein kinase (DMPK) gene on chromosome 19q13.2. The anticipation phenomenon is caused by expansion of the mutation size from one generation to the next. The disease involves the gastrointestinal tract, respiratory and cardiac muscle, the eyes, and endocrine function. Affected patients may also have neurobehavioral abnormalities. Life expectancy is greatly reduced.[30]

In a review of 31 women with DM1 with 78 pregnancies, only 16% knew their diagnosis before contemplating their first pregnancy and many had obstetric complications. Although early miscarriages occurred at a rate similar to that of the general population, late spontaneous abortions were seen in 4% of woman who were symptomatic. Increased risk of ectopic pregnancy (4% of all gestations) was thought to be related to fallopian tube smooth muscle dysfunction. Risk of abnormal implantation and urinary tract infections was increased. Preterm labor before 34 weeks occurred in 19% of gestations, often with congenitally affected infants. Labor abnormalities of all 3 stages were frequent and operative deliveries were increased at 36%. Increased perinatal death was seen (up to 15%) mainly in infants affected by congenital DM during pregnancy. Most women postnatally return to their prepregnancy functional capacity; pregnancy does not seem to have a significant impact on the course of maternal disease.[66]

Myotonic dystrophy type 2 (DM2), or proximal myotonic myopathy (PROMM), is an autosomal dominant multisystem disorder whose clinical manifestations resemble DM1. Anticipation is less prominent than in DM1 and a congenital form has not been described.[30] Retrospective data from 96 pregnancies in 42 women suggest that pregnancy may hasten the onset or progression of DM2. Women with prior pregnancies had onset of symptoms at an earlier age than the general population of men and women with DM2.

The disease may affect pregnancy in some with DM2, although rates of miscarriage, perinatal death, or other fetal risk are not increased for the group as a whole. If onset of symptoms occurs before or during pregnancy, there is a higher rate of preterm labor, prematurity, and fetal loss. When onset or worsening of symptoms occurs during pregnancy, patients generally improve after delivery. This group has similar worsening in subsequent pregnancies.[67]

Nondystrophic Myotonias and Periodic Paralysis

Myotonia congenita (MC) and paramyotonia congenita (PMC) are muscle channelopathies that result in electrical myotonia; however, the muscle tissues are not dystrophic.[30] There are case reports of myotonia worsening during pregnancy in MC and PMC. Avoidance of precipitants of myotonia, including cold temperatures, is recommended. No adverse effect on labor, delivery, or infant outcome has been reported.[68,69]

Congenital Nemaline Rod Myopathy

Congenital nemaline rod myopathy is a slowly progressive inherited myopathy characterized by smooth and skeletal muscle weakness, hypotonia, and skeletal deformities. Facial abnormalities including retrognathia, micrognathia, prognathism, high arched palate, rare cardiac involvement, and restrictive lung disease pose challenges during labor and general anesthesia. Bone deformities, contractures, lordosis, and kyphosis can complicate regional anesthesia. Spontaneous vaginal deliveries have been reported in nemaline myopathy with uncomplicated pregnancies. The method of delivery should be individualized based on disease severity.[70,71]

Women with several muscles diseases, including King syndrome,[72] multiminicore myopathy, central core disease,[73] and Native American myopathy (NAM),[74] have an increased incidence of malignant hyperthermia (MH). During delivery, halogenated inhaled anesthetics and succinylcholine must be avoided and patients require close monitoring. Dantrolene can be used to treat MH associated with cesarean section but it is debated whether to use dantrolene prophylactically because it can cause muscle weakness and uterine atony in the mother.[72] Uneventful pregnancy with vaginal delivery[75] and successful vaginal delivery with an epidural of ropivacaine[76] in the same patient with multiminicore myopathy have been reported.

Metabolic Myopathy

Primary metabolic myopathies (MM) are inherited and classified by their underlying biochemical abnormalities as disorders of carbohydrate, lipid, and adenine nucleotide metabolism or associated mitochondrial encephalomyopathies. These disorders are characterized by fixed, progressive weakness and/or weakness induced by exercise.[30] Secondary MM can occur because of electrolyte abnormalities, endocrinopathies, and certain drugs. Isolated cases in pregnancy have been reported.

Myophosphorylase deficiency (McArdle disease) is the most common disorder of carbohydrate metabolism. It is autosomal recessive, characterized by exercise intolerance, and presents in children and young adults.[30] Pregnancy is generally unaffected by the disease.[77,78] One affected woman had an episode of exercise-induced myoglobinuria and increase in her serum CK in the first trimester. Her pregnancy was otherwise uncomplicated and she delivered via cesarean section for malposition of the fetal head.[77] In a review of anesthesia for patients with McArdle disease, 3 women underwent cesarean section both with general and epidural anesthesia without complication. Although there is a potential risk of perioperative fatigue, myoglobinuria, and renal failure, few problems generally arise. There was no clinical incidence of MH. It is recommended that precautions be taken to prevent muscle ischemia and rhabdomyolysis.[79] Myoadenylate deaminase (MADA) is an isoenzyme of the adenosine monophosphate deaminase (AMPD) found in skeletal muscle. This disorder of nucleotide metabolism is characterized by exertional pain, fatigue, and possible myoglobinuria in late adolescence to middle age.[30] Two pregnancies in 1 patient with myoadenylate deaminase deficiency myopathy have been reported. Both resulted in uncomplicated vaginal deliveries of healthy infants.[80]

Hypokalemic periodic paralysis can be exacerbated by high-carbohydrate diets, glucose and insulin infusions, cold, stress, alcohol, β-agonists, and other medications that cause intracellular shift of potassium. Cases in pregnancy have been reported after betamethasone injections,[81] as a presentation of hyperthyroidism,[82] after a 1-hour glucose tolerance test,[83] and after excessive caffeine consumption.[84] Pregnancy and anesthesia can precipitate attacks of familial hypokalemic periodic paralysis (FHPP). Avoidance of intravenous glucose, potassium supplementation, early epidural analgesia, and a passive second stage of labor may help avoid a paralytic episode.[85] Andersen-Tawil syndrome (ATS) is hereditary periodic paralysis associated with cardiac abnormalities. There is 1 reported case of pregnancy in a woman with ATS with a successful term birth.[86]

Hypokalemic myopathy has been reported in pregnancy from pica of clay[87] and baking soda.[88] Symptoms ranged from myalgias, mild weakness, and fatigue to hypokalemic metabolic alkalosis, rhabdomyolysis, increase in serum transaminases, and hypertension. All symptoms resolved within days after potassium supplementation and discontinuation of the nonfood material.[88]

MITOCHONDRIAL MYOPATHY

Although mitochondrial myopathies are a rare and diverse group of metabolic defects in the physiology of the mitochondrial respiratory chain, several successful pregnancies have been reported. There is no consensus about the best mode of delivery.[89–91] Magnesium may interfere with calcium-dependent enzymes in the respiratory chain and should be avoided.[19]

One pregnancy was reported in a woman with mitochondrial thymidine kinase 2 deficiency and chronic respiratory failure requiring noninvasive positive pressure ventilation (NIPPV) because of severe neuromuscular weakness. Pregnancy was complicated by increased dependence on NIPPV during pregnancy and multiple episodes of preeclampsia. She had preterm birth via cesarean section with an epidural and continued NIPPV. The infant was healthy when discharged at day 28.[92]

Mitochondrial myopathy, encephalopathy, lactic acidosis, and strokelike episodes (MELAS) syndrome can cause neuromuscular, metabolic, cardiac, gastrointestinal, cognitive, and hepatic dysfunction. The disease can affect skeletal and cardiac muscle. The course of pregnancy in these patients reflects the phenotypic variability of the disease. Uncomplicated pregnancies and spontaneous vaginal deliveries of healthy infants have been reported in patients with mild disease.[93] Pregnancy may also be complicated by heart failure with acute pulmonary edema and fetal loss [94] or status epilepticus.[95] Specific strategies and an interdisciplinary evaluation to minimize metabolic demands are recommended to avoid acidosis during labor and delivery.[93]

Carnitine palmitoyltransferase 1 (CPT1) deficiency is a disorder of mitochondrial fatty acid β-oxidation with autosomal recessive inheritance. A woman with previously undiagnosed disease had a pregnancy complicated by hemolysis, increased liver enzymes, low platelets (HELLP) syndrome but gave birth to a healthy infant.[96] Carnitine controls the influx of long-chain fatty acids into mitochondria and contributes to muscular energy supply. Carnitine deficiency myopathy is characterized pathologically by abnormal lipid storage with or without necrosis and ragged red fibers. It can be seen secondary to genetic defects of intermediary metabolism, especially mitochondrial respiratory chain defects, β-oxidation enzyme defects, or drug therapy causing progressive weakness with an increased serum CK. In healthy individuals, plasma carnitine levels are reduced at the end of pregnancy and return to baseline after a month postpartum. Women with carnitine deficiency cannot effectively replete muscle carnitine from plasma supplies. Pregnancy and the postpartum period may unmask a latent carnitine deficiency or worsen an existing myopathy.[90] Symptoms may improve or stabilize with carnitine supplementation. Patients with carnitine deficiency isolated to muscle may improve more with supplementation than patients with systemic carnitine deficiency.[90,91]

MOTOR NEURON DISEASE
Spinal Muscular Atrophy

The Spinal muscular atrophies (SMAs) are progressive, phenotypically heterogeneous hereditary diseases of anterior horn cells and motor cranial nerve nuclei. They are characterized based on phenotype including age of onset, life expectancy, and the milestones achieved.[30] Onset can occur during infancy or adulthood. The course and outcome of pregnancy and possible effects on muscle weakness, examined in 12 patients with SMA during 17 pregnancies, showed that 80% of patients experienced complications during pregnancy, including preterm labor. No adverse effects on the development of the infants were noted. Eight patients had worsening weakness in the second trimester and 5 noted persistence of their deterioration after pregnancy. The age of onset or the clinical course of the disease did not predict deterioration during pregnancy.

Multidisciplinary planning is necessary before delivery because of potential respiratory compromise, airway difficulties, and spinal column deformity. Cesarean section is the most common method of delivery but patients with less disease burden have adequate uterine function and can deliver vaginally. General anesthesia is used with caution because of restriction in mouth opening, sensitivity to muscle relaxants, and hyperkalemia after administration of some paralytics.[97] Successful use of dexmedetomidine for awake fiberoptic intubation[98] and subarachnoid block for elective cesarean section[99] are reported.

Amyotrophic Lateral Sclerosis

Amyotrophic lateral sclerosis (ALS) is a disorder of widespread degeneration of upper and lower motor neurons. Although 90% to 95% of cases are sporadic, it may be inherited in an autosomal dominant, x-linked recessive or mitochondrial pattern. The incidence is 1.8/100,000, with an average age of onset of 60 years. Women are affected twice as often as men; however, this gender difference disappears in postmenopausal women.[30] Among 13 cases published in the English language since 1977, 8 patients were diagnosed during pregnancy.[100] Pregnancy may limit maternal survival and reduce maternal quality of life, but it is not clear that ALS causes obstetric complications. In this group, no deaths were reported caused by neurologic complications. However, some women had rapid progression, respiratory failure, percutaneous endoscopic gastrostomy (PEG) tube and tracheotomy placement. Three patients died postpartum. One had a therapeutic abortion caused by worsening dyspnea, 5 delivered preterm, and 4 required cesarean section. There were no neonatal complications.[101]

The effect of pregnancy may depend on disease severity. One woman with sporadic ALS became pregnant twice, 13 and 28 months after the onset of symptoms. Before her second pregnancy, she was bedridden. The first pregnancy resulted in the vaginal delivery of a healthy baby without complications. During her second pregnancy she required a PEG tube, cesarean section at 34 weeks, and the infant required artificial ventilation in an intensive care unit for 72 hours. The patient underwent tracheostomy and required ventilation 2 months later, and died after 9 months.[102] Anticipatory counseling and early discussions about invasive ventilation are recommended in women of childbearing age.

Riluzole, a glutamate antagonist, is the only FDA-approved medication for the treatment of ALS. There have been no adequate human studies of the effect in pregnancy. It is unknown whether riluzole is excreted in breast milk. Preclinical studies showed embryotoxicity, impaired male and female fertility, increased intrauterine death, and reduced offspring viability in doses from 1.5 to 11 times the normal human recommended dose. The FDA classified the medication as category C.[103] One woman who took riluzole at a standard 100 mg/d dose for the duration of her pregnancy is reported. She had a normal term vaginal delivery. The infant developed normally through follow-up at 1 year.[100]

CLINICAL CASE STUDY

An otherwise-healthy 26-year-old woman was seen as an inpatient 2 days postpartum. Over the previous year, she had noticed generalized fatigue. In the final month of pregnancy, she developed intermittent ptosis and diplopia, chewing fatigue, dysphagia, and upper extremity weakness. She delivered a healthy term infant via a forceps-assisted vaginal delivery. The infant was later transferred to the special care nursery with feeding difficulties and mild generalized weakness.

The patient's physical examination was notable for weakness of eye closure, cheek puff, neck flexion, shoulder abduction, finger extension, and hip flexion. Fatigable ptosis and binocular diplopia referable to the medial rectus muscles were present. Electrodiagnostic evaluation was notable for a 25% decrement with 3-Hz repetitive nerve stimulation of the spinal accessory nerve recording over the trapezius. Acetylcholine receptor binding antibodies were subsequently positive at 34.5 nmol/L (negative ≤0.02 nmol/L). Chest computed tomography revealed no evidence of thymoma. Thyroid function testing was normal. She was diagnosed with seropositive, generalized MG. Before discharge, she received a course of plasma exchange with significant improvement in her weakness. Prednisone 60 mg by mouth daily and Mestinon 30 mg by mouth 3 times a day as needed were initiated.

She had sustained improvement in her strength over the next 8 months and underwent thymectomy without complication or worsening weakness. Pathology revealed benign fibrovascular and adipose tissue. Over 2 years, prednisone was gradually tapered to 12.5 mg by mouth every other day. At this dose, she experienced worsening weakness and had another course of plasma exchange. Mycophenolate mofetil and azathioprine were considered; however, because she was planning another pregnancy, neither medication was initiated. Prednisone was increased to 20 mg daily and she was counseled to postpone pregnancy until she had shown lasting improvement in her strength. She was referred to the maternal fetal medicine clinic to establish care. Over the next 7 months, she was able to taper her prednisone to 30 mg by mouth every other day with minimal manifestations of MG.

At her next follow-up appointment, she was pregnant and in the first trimester. This pregnancy was complicated by gestational diabetes; however, her MG remained stable. She delivered a healthy infant at 39 weeks via a spontaneous vaginal delivery with epidural anesthesia. She had transient diplopia in the immediate postpartum period in the setting of sleep deprivation. Prednisone was continued with the plan to taper her dose if she remained stable for 6 months postpartum.

Comment

This patient's history and initial examination showed fluctuating, fatigable ocular, bulbar, and limb weakness that presented in the third trimester of pregnancy. She came to medical attention in the immediate postpartum period with worsening symptoms and when weakness was noted in her newborn. Her presentation, electro-diagnostic studies, and acetylcholine receptor antibody status were consistent with acquired seropositive generalized MG. Because of her degree of weakness and potential for further worsening in the postpartum period, plasma exchange and corti-costeroids were initiated immediately after diagnosis. Her newborn was affected by transient neonatal MG. The infant required supportive care and cholinesterase inhib-itors for 10 days until symptoms resolved.

She was followed frequently in pregnancy and the postpartum period. The goal of treatment was to achieve minimal manifestations of MG on therapy without significant teratogenic potential before her second pregnancy. Once she passed the postpartum period, thymectomy was performed before her next pregnancy to help her achieve the best chance for long-term disease remission on minimal or no immunosuppression. As this case shows, the course of MG in one pregnancy does not predict its course in subsequent pregnancies. A collaborative approach with other specialties is essen-tial from the time of planning pregnancy to the postpartum period.

SUMMARY

How to counsel and treat women with neuromuscular disorders before and during pregnancy is based on limited data from case reports and retrospective studies of patients with heterogeneous disease. For each patient, the approach should be gener-ated by an interdisciplinary team of physicians and based on the individual's current manifestations and history of disease. If there are genetic implications for the offspring, genetic counseling is recommended. The medical team must be cautious to present a realistic picture of the data that are known and what remains unknown. For some women with neuromuscular disorders, the impact of pregnancy on their disease and the effect of their disease on their pregnancy may be significant and longstanding. Others, even when severely affected, have achieved successful pregnancies and deliv-eries without significant complications.

REFERENCES

1. Padua L, Pasquale AD, Pazzaglia C, et al. Systematic review of pregnancy-related carpal tunnel syndrome. Muscle Nerve 2010;42(5):697–702.
2. Stewart JD. Focal peripheral neuropathies. 3rd edition. Philadelphia: Lippincott Williams & Wilkins; 2000. p. 211–13, 457–66, 475–8.
3. Mondelli M, Rossi S, Monti E, et al. Prospective study of positive factors for improvement of carpal tunnel syndrome in pregnant women. Muscle Nerve 2007;36(6):778–83.
4. Padua L, Aprile I, Caliandro P, et al. Symptoms and neurophysiological picture of carpal tunnel syndrome in pregnancy. Clin Neurophysiol 2001;112(10): 1946–51.
5. Turgut F, Cetinsahin M, Bolukbasi O. The management of carpal tunnel syndrome in pregnancy. J Clin Neurosci 2001;8(4):332–4.
6. Wand J. Carpal tunnel syndrome in pregnancy and lactation. J Hand Surg Br 1990;15(1):93–5.
7. Padua L, Aprile I, Caliandro P, et al. Carpal tunnel syndrome in pregnancy. Neurology 2002;59(10):1643.
8. Baumann F, Karlikaya G, Yuksel G. The subclinical incidence of CTS in preg-nancy: assessment of median nerve impairment in asymptomatic pregnant women. Neurol Neurophysiol Neurosci 2007;3:1–8.

9. Kaplan Y, Kurt S, Karaer H. Carpal tunnel syndrome in postmenopausal women. J Neurol Sci 2008;270(1-2):77–81.
10. Wong C, Scavone B, Dugan S, et al. Incidence of postpartum lumbosacral spine and lower extremity nerve injuries. Obstet Gynecol 2003;101(2):279–88.
11. Van Diver T, Camann W. Meralgia paresthetica in the parturient. Int J Obstet Anesth 1995;4(2):109–12.
12. Devers A, Galer B. Topical lidocaine patch relieves a variety of neuropathic pain conditions: an open-label study. Clin J Pain 2000;16(3):205–8.
13. United States Food and Drug Administration (FDA). Department of Health and Human Services. Subchapter C–Drugs: General. Code of Federal Regulations. Title 21, vol. 4. Revised as of April 1, 2011. Available at: http://www.accessdata.fda.gov/scripts/cdrh/cfdocs/cfCFR/CFRSearch.cfm?CFRPart=201&showFR=1. Accessed May 22, 2012.
14. LaBan M, Rapp N, Oeyen von P. The lumbar herniated disk of pregnancy: a report of six cases identified by magnetic resonance imaging. Arch Phys Med Rehabil 1995;76:476–9.
15. Ng J, Kitchen N. Neurosurgery and pregnancy. J Neurol Neurosurg Psychiatr 2008;79(7):745–52.
16. Chen M, Coakley F, Kaimal A. Guidelines for computed tomography and magnetic resonance imaging use during pregnancy and lactation. Obstet Gynecol 2008;112:333–40.
17. Carette S, Fehlings MG. Clinical practice. Cervical radiculopathy. N Engl J Med 2005;353(4):392–9.
18. Chow J, Chen K, Sen R, et al. Cauda equina syndrome post-caesarean section. Aust N Z J Obstet Gynaecol 2008;48(2):218–20.
19. Sax TW, Rosenbaum RB. Neuromuscular disorders in pregnancy. Muscle Nerve 2006;34(5):559–71.
20. Hakim al M, Katirji B. Femoral mononeuropathy induced by the lithotomy position - a report of 5 cases with a review of literature. Muscle Nerve 1993;16(9):891–5.
21. Cohen Y, Lavie O, Granovsky-Grisaru S, et al. Bell's palsy complicating pregnancy: a review. Obstet Gynecol Surv 2000;55(3):184–8.
22. Gillman G, Schaitkin B, May M, et al. Bell's palsy in pregnancy: a study of recovery outcomes. Otolaryngol Head Neck Surg 2002;126(1):26–30.
23. Katz A, Sergienko R, Dior U, et al. Bell's palsy during pregnancy: is it associated with adverse perinatal outcome? Laryngoscope 2011;121(7):1395–8.
24. Robinson J, Pou J. Bell's palsy: a predisposition of pregnant women. Arch Otolaryngol 1972;95:125–9.
25. Shmorgun D, Chan W-S, Ray JG. Association between Bell's palsy in pregnancy and pre-eclampsia. QJM 2002;95(6):359–62.
26. Roubal P, Chavinson A, LaGrandeur R. Bilateral radial nerve palsies from use of the standard birthing bar. Obstet Gynecol 1996;87(5):820–1.
27. Skeen MB, Eggleston M. Thoraconeuralgia gravidarum. Muscle Nerve 1999;22(6):779–80.
28. Pleet AB, Massey E. Intercostal neuralgia of pregnancy. JAMA 1980;243(8):770.
29. Samlaska S, Dews T. Long-term epidural analgesia for pregnancy-induced intercostal neuralgia. Pain 1995;62(2):245–8.
30. Amato AA, Russell JA. Neuromuscular disorders. New York (NY): McGraw-Hill; 2008. p. 97–9, 123, 161, 213–15, 233, 552–3, 597, 604, 609, 647–50, 655.
31. Chan LY, Tsui MH, Leung TN. Guillain-Barré syndrome in pregnancy. Acta Obstet Gynecol Scand 2004;83(4):319–25.

32. Rees J, Soudain S, Gregson N. *Campylobacter jejuni* infection and Guillain-Barré syndrome. N Engl J Med 1995;333:1374–9.
33. Wiertlewski S, Magot A, Drapier S, et al. Worsening of neurologic symptoms after epidural anesthesia for labor in a Guillain-Barre patient. Anesth Analg 2004;98(3):825–7.
34. McCombe PA, McManis PG, Frith JA, et al. Chronic inflammatory demyelinating polyradiculoneuropathy associated with pregnancy. Ann Neurol 1987;21(1):102–4.
35. Cats EA, Jacobs BC, Yuki N, et al. Multifocal motor neuropathy: association of anti-GM1 IgM antibodies with clinical features. Neurology 2010;75(22):1961–7.
36. Chaudhry V, Escolar DM, Cornblath DR. Worsening of multifocal motor neuropathy during pregnancy. Neurology 2002;59(1):139–41.
37. Attarian S, Azulay JP, Chabrol B, et al. Neonatal lower motor neuron syndrome associated with maternal neuropathy with anti-GM1 IgG. Neurology 2004;63(2):379–81.
38. Váncsa A, Ponyi A, Constantin T, et al. Pregnancy outcome in idiopathic inflammatory myopathy. Rheumatol Int 2006;27(5):435–9.
39. Silva C, Sultan S, Isenberg D. Pregnancy outcome in adult-onset idiopathic inflammatory myopathy. Rheumatology 2003;42(10):1168–72.
40. Williams L, Chang PY, Park E, et al. Successful treatment of dermatomyositis during pregnancy with intravenous immunoglobulin monotherapy. Obstet Gynecol 2007;109(2 Pt 2):561–3.
41. Mosca M, Strigini F, Carmignani A, et al. Pregnant patient with dermatomyositis successfully treated with intravenous immunoglobulin therapy. Arthritis Rheum 2005;53(1):119–21.
42. Messina S, Fagiolari G, Lamperti C, et al. Women with pregnancy-related polymyositis and high serum CK levels in the newborn. Neurology 2002;58(3):482–4.
43. Batocchi A, Majolini L, Evoli A, et al. Course and treatment of myasthenia gravis during pregnancy. Neurology 1999;52:447.
44. Ciafaloni E, Massey J. Myasthenia gravis and pregnancy. Neurol Clin 2004;22(4):771.
45. Wen JC, Liu TC, Chen YH, et al. No increased risk of adverse pregnancy outcomes for women with myasthenia gravis: a nationwide population-based study. Eur J Neurol 2009;16(8):889–94.
46. Djelmis J, Sostarko M, Mayer D, et al. Myasthenia gravis in pregnancy: report on 69 cases. Eur J Obstet Gynecol Reprod Biol 2002;104(1):21–5.
47. American Academy of Pediatrics Committee on Drugs. Transfer of drugs and other chemicals into human milk. Pediatrics 2001;108(3):776–89.
48. Hoff J, Daltveit A, Gilhus N. Myasthenia gravis. Neurology 2003;61(10):1362.
49. Kuczkowski KM. Labor analgesia for the parturient with neurological disease: what does an obstetrician need to know? Arch Gynecol Obstet 2006;274(1):41–6.
50. Bashuk RG, Krendel DA. Myasthenia gravis presenting as weakness after magnesium administration. Muscle Nerve 1990;13(8):708–12.
51. Ahlsten G, Lefvert AK, Osterman PO, et al. Follow-up study of muscle function in children of mothers with myasthenia gravis during pregnancy. J Child Neurol 1992;7(3):264–9.
52. Oskoui M, Jacobson L, Chung WK, et al. Fetal acetylcholine receptor inactivation syndrome and maternal myasthenia gravis. Neurology 2008;71(24):2010–2.
53. Niks EH, Verrips A, Semmekrot BA, et al. A transient neonatal myasthenic syndrome with anti-MUSK antibodies. Neurology 2008;70(14):1215–6.

54. Hoff JM, Daltveit AK, Gilhus NE. Myasthenia gravis in pregnancy and birth: identifying risk factors, optimising care. Eur J Neurol 2007;14(1):38–43.
55. Schneider-Gold C, Wessig C, Höpker M, et al. Pregnancy and delivery of a healthy baby in autoimmune Lambert-Eaton myasthenic syndrome. J Neurol 2006;253(9):1236–7.
56. Reuner U, Kamin G, Ramantani G, et al. Transient neonatal Lambert-Eaton syndrome. J Neurol 2008;255(11):1827–8.
57. Hoff JM, Gilhus NE, Daltveit AK. Pregnancies and deliveries in patients with Charcot-Marie-Tooth disease. Neurology 2005;64(3):459–62.
58. Rudnik-Schöneborn S, Röhrig D, Nicholson G, et al. Pregnancy and delivery in Charcot-Marie-Tooth disease type 1. Neurology 1993;43(10):2011.
59. Simonetti S. Lesion of the anterior branch of axillary nerve in a patient with hereditary neuropathy with liability to pressure palsies. Eur J Neurol 2000;7(5): 577–9.
60. Peters G, Hinds NP. Inherited neuropathy can cause postpartum foot drop. Anesth Analg 2005;100(2):547–8.
61. Stögbauer F, Young P, Kuhlenbäumer G, et al. Hereditary recurrent focal neuropathies. Neurology 2000;54(3):546.
62. van Alfen N, van Engelen B. The clinical spectrum of neuralgic amyotrophy in 246 cases. Brain 2006;129(2):438–50.
63. Klein C, Dyck P, Friedenberg S, et al. Inflammation and neuropathic attacks in hereditary brachial plexus neuropathy. J Neurol Neurosurg Psychiatr 2002; 73(1):45.
64. Ciafaloni E, Pressman EK, Loi AM, et al. Pregnancy and birth outcomes in women with facioscapulohumeral muscular dystrophy. Neurology 2006;67(10): 1887–9.
65. Rudnik-Schoneborn S, Glauner B, Rohrig D, et al. Obstetric aspects in women with facioscapulohumeral muscular dystrophy, limb-girdle muscular dystrophy, and congenital myopathies. Arch Neurol 1997;54(7):888.
66. Rudnik-Schöneborn S, Zerres K. Outcome in pregnancies complicated by myotonic dystrophy: a study of 31 patients and review of the literature. Eur J Obstet Gynecol Reprod Biol 2004;114(1):44–53.
67. Rudnik-Schoneborn S, Schneider-Gold C, Raabe U, et al. Outcome and effect of pregnancy in myotonic dystrophy type 2. Neurology 2006;66(4):579–80.
68. Chitayat D, Etchell M, Wilson RD. Cold-induced abortion in paramyotonia congenita. Am J Obstet Gynecol 1988;158(2):435–6.
69. Lacomis D, Gonzales J, Giuliani M. Fluctuating clinical myotonia and weakness from Thomsen's disease occurring only during pregnancies. Clin Neurol Neurosurg 1999;101(2):133–6.
70. Eskandar O, Eckford S. Pregnancy in a patient with nemaline myopathy. Obstet Gynecol 2007;109:501–4.
71. Stackhouse R, Chelmow D. Anesthetic complications in a pregnant patient with nemaline myopathy. Anesth Analg 1994;79:1195–7.
72. Habib AS, Millar S, Deballi P, et al. Anesthetic management of a ventilator-dependent parturient with the King-Denborough syndrome. Can J Anaesth 2003;50(6):589–92.
73. Robinson R, Carpenter D, Shaw MA, et al. Mutations in RYR1in malignant hyperthermia and central core disease. Hum Mutat 2006;27(10):977–89.
74. Stamm DS, Powell CM, Stajich JM, et al. Novel congenital myopathy locus identified in Native American Indians at 12q13.13-14.1. Neurology 2008;71(22): 1764–9.

75. Osada H, Masuda K, Seki K, et al. Multi-minicore disease with susceptibility to malignant hyperthermia in pregnancy. Gynecol Obstet Invest 2004;58(1):32–5.
76. Saito O, Yamamoto T, Mizuno Y. Epidural anesthetic management using ropivacaine in a parturient with multi-minicore disease and susceptibility to malignant hyperthermia. J Anesth 2007;21(1):113.
77. Giles W, Maher C. Myophosphorylase deficiency (McArdle disease) in a patient with normal pregnancy and normal pregnancy outcome. Obstet Med 2011;4(3): 120–1.
78. Cochrane P, Alderman B. Normal pregnancy and successful delivery in myophosphorylase deficiency (McArdle's disease). J Neurol 1973;36:225–7.
79. Bollig G, Mohr S, Raeder J. McArdle's disease and anaesthesia: case reports. Review of potential problems and association with malignant hyperthermia. Acta Anaesthesiol Scand 2005;49(8):1077–83.
80. Bellver J, Cervera J, Boldó A, et al. Myoadenylate deaminase deficiency myopathy in pregnancy. Arch Gynecol Obstet 1997;259(3):157–9.
81. Teagarden CM, Picardo CW. Betamethasone-induced hypokalemic periodic paralysis in pregnancy. Obstet Gynecol 2011;117(2 Pt 2):433–5.
82. Donovan L, Parkins VM, Mahalingham A. Thyrotoxic periodic paralysis in pregnancy with impaired glucose tolerance: a case report and discussion of management issues. Thyroid 2007;17(6):579–83.
83. Damallie KK, Drake JG, Block WA. Hypokalemic periodic paralysis in pregnancy after 1-hour glucose screen. Obstet Gynecol 2000;95(6 Pt 2):1037.
84. Appel C, Myles T. Caffeine-induced hypokalemic paralysis in pregnancy. Obstet Gynecol 2001;97(5):805–7.
85. Viscomi C, Ptacek L, Dudley D. Anesthetic management of familial hypokalemic periodic paralysis during parturition. Anesth Analg 1999;88(5):1081.
86. Subbiah RN, Gula LJ, Skanes AC, et al. Andersen-Tawil syndrome: management challenges during pregnancy, labor, and delivery. J Cardiovasc Electrophysiol 2008;19(9):987–9.
87. Ukaonu C, Hill A, Christensen F. Hypokalemic myopathy in pregnancy caused by clay ingestion. Obstet Gynecol 2003;102(5):1169–71.
88. Grotegut C, Dandolu V, Katari S. Baking soda pica: a case of hypokalemic metabolic alkalosis and rhabdomyolysis in pregnancy. Obstet Gynecol 2006;107(2): 484–6.
89. Blake L, Shaw R. Mitochondrial myopathy in a primigravid pregnancy. Br J Obstet Gynaecol 1999;106:871–3.
90. Koller H, Stoll G, Neuen-Jacob E. Postpartum manifestation of a necrotising lipid storage myopathy associated with muscle carnitine deficiency. J Neurol Neurosurg Psychiatr 1998;64(3):407–8.
91. Angelini C, Govoni E, Bragaglia MM, et al. Carnitine deficiency: acute postpartum crisis. Ann Neurol 1978;4(6):558–61.
92. Yuan N, El-Sayed YY, Ruoss SJ, et al. Successful pregnancy and cesarean delivery via noninvasive ventilation in mitochondrial myopathy. J Perinatol 2009; 29(2):166–7.
93. Maurtua M, Torres A, Ibarra V, et al. Anesthetic management of an obstetric patient with MELAS syndrome: case report and literature review. Int J Obstet Anesth 2008;17(4):370–3.
94. Sánchez MV, Romero R. Acute pulmonary edema secondary to pregnancy in a patient with the mitochondrial disease MELAS. Rev Esp Cardiol 2010;63(5):615–7.
95. Sikdar S, Sahni V, Miglani A, et al. Pregnancy-precipitated status epilepticus: a rare presentation of MELAS syndrome. Neurol India 2007;55(1):82.

96. Ylitalo K, Vänttinen T, Halmesmäki E, et al. Serious pregnancy complications in a patient with previously undiagnosed carnitine palmitoyltransferase 1 deficiency. Am J Obstet Gynecol 2005;192(6):2060–2.

97. Flunt D, Andreadis N, Menadue C, et al. Clinical commentary: obstetric and respiratory management of pregnancy with severe spinal muscular atrophy. Obstet Gynecol Int 2009;2009:1–5.

98. Neumann MM, Davio MB, Macknet MR, et al. Dexmedetomidine for awake fiber-optic intubation in a parturient with spinal muscular atrophy type III for cesarean delivery. Int J Obstet Anesth 2009;18(4):403–7.

99. Harris S, Moaz K. Caesarean section conducted under subarachnoid block in two sisters with spinal muscular atrophy. Int J Obstet Anesth 2002;11(2):125–7.

100. Kawamichi Y, Makino Y, Matsuda Y, et al. Riluzole use during pregnancy in a patient with amyotrophic lateral sclerosis: a case report. J Int Med Res 2010;38(2):720–6.

101. Chiò A, Calvo A, Di Vito N, et al. Amyotrophic lateral sclerosis associated with pregnancy: report of four new cases and review of the literature. Amyotroph Lateral Scler Other Motor Neuron Disord 2003;4(1):45–8.

102. Sarafov S, Doitchinova M, Karagiozova Z, et al. Two consecutive pregnancies in early and late stage of amyotrophic lateral sclerosis. Amyotroph Lateral Scler 2009;10(5-6):483–6.

103. FDA. Rilutek (riluzole) Tablets. 2009. Available at: http://www.accessdata.fda. gov/drugsatfda_docs/label/2009/020599s011s012lbl.pdf. Accessed October 16, 2011.

Stroke and Pregnancy

Barbara Tettenborn, MD, PhD[a,b]

KEYWORDS

- Cerebrovascular disease • Stroke • Pregnancy • Puerperium • Hemorrhage
- Cerebral ischemia

KEY POINTS

- Strategies for stroke prevention should take into account the competing risks to mother and fetus.
- Treatment of acute stroke in pregnant women is still controversial, but not strictly contraindicated.
- Several case reports have documented successful reperfusion, in addition to satisfactory maternal and fetal outcomes.
- Aspirin and warfarin are considered safe in the second and third trimesters.
- There are no trials of anticoagulation or antiplatelet therapies of stroke prevention in pregnancy.

INTRODUCTION

Stroke is an important contributor to maternal morbidity and mortality. It is reported that 12% to 35% of cerebrovascular disease in those aged 15 to 45 years involved either pregnancy or recent delivery.[1,2] Cerebrovascular events in pregnancy are divided into ischemic and hemorrhagic disorders. Ischemic disorders are characterized by insufficient blood flow to a particular area in the brain, whereas, in hemorrhages, blood extravasates into brain parenchyma or the subarachnoid space. Pregnancy and the postpartum period are associated with an increased risk of ischemic stroke and cerebral hemorrhage but few studies exist on this topic and the estimates of incidence vary widely in epidemiologic studies from 4.3 to 210 per 100,000 deliveries. The disparity between estimates is attributed to different study designs, patient group selection, inadequate consideration of referral bias, and small sample size. Recent studies from the United States that included a large number of patients report a risk of stroke of 13.1 to 29.1 per 100,000 deliveries.[1–3] Kuklina and colleagues[4] analyzed the hospital discharge data from the US Nationwide Inpatient

The author has nothing to disclose.
[a] Department of Neurology, Kantonsspital St. Gallen, CH-9007 Street Gallen, Switzerland;
[b] University of Mainz, D-55131 Mainz, Germany
E-mail address: barbara.tettenborn@kssg.ch

Sample regarding pregnancy-related hospitalizations that have involved a stroke. The results showed an increasing trend in the rate of pregnancy-related hospitalizations with stroke in the United States, especially during the postpartum period, from 1994/1995 to 2006/2007. Data exist from the Shanghai Women's Health Study, a large population-based cohort study of almost 75,000 Chinese women, that high gravidity or parity may be related to increased risk of stroke in women.[5]

Several physiologic and pathophysiologic changes during pregnancy make the cause of both ischemia and hemorrhage different from those in nonpregnant women. For a long time, especially before the advent of computed tomography (CT) and magnetic resonance imaging (MRI), it was thought that most strokes in pregnancy were attributable to cerebral venous and sinus thrombosis, but many recent studies indicate that arterial ischemic strokes are equally or more prevalent than venous infarcts. The differentiation of stroke causes has been made easier by advanced neuroimaging techniques, but the question of cause still represents a challenge.

RISK FACTORS FOR STROKE IN PREGNANCY AND PUERPERIUM

Pregnant women may have risk factors that are typically associated with stroke in the general population (eg, hypertension, cigarette smoking, diabetes, valvular heart disease, hypercoagulable disorders), and this may be especially important with the increasing prevalence of obesity at younger age and increasing maternal age. Hypertension in pregnancy might be preexisting, gestational, or associated with preeclampsia or eclampsia. In contrast, there are several physiologic changes that occur during pregnancy that may predispose to cerebrovascular disease, such as endocrine, metabolic, and cardiovascular changes.

Skilton and colleagues[6] recently published the results of their study on 1005 women and 781 men regarding the association of childbearing, child rearing, cardiovascular risk factors, and progression of carotid intima-media thickness over a 6-year follow-up period. For women, childbirth during the 6-year follow-up was associated with concurrent reductions in high-density lipoprotein cholesterol, apolipoprotein A-I and apolipoprotein B, a redistribution of adiposity to abdominal deposits, and increased progression of carotid intima-media thickness. This association of childbirth with carotid intima-media thickness progression was not greatly modified by adjustment for concurrent changes in cardiovascular risk factors. The association was significantly stronger in women than in men, who served as a control group exposed to the social and lifestyle influences of child rearing but not the biologic influences of childbearing. These findings provide evidence that childbearing can have a rapid influence on the progression of atherosclerosis. This influence is only partially mediated by changes in cardiovascular risk factors, suggesting that some proportion of the association is caused by unidentified mechanisms, possibly including a short-term influence of pregnancy itself.

TIMING OF STROKE CAUSED BY PHYSIOLOGIC CHANGES IN PREGNANCY

Physiologic changes in pregnancy affect almost every organ and system and make the risk of stroke higher toward the end of pregnancy because of constantly increasing estrogen and progesterone levels making the risk of stroke higher because of the increasing production of clotting factors by estrogen, venous dilation by progesterone, and increasing water retention. Postpartum, the rapid decrease in the level of progesterone may provoke vasoconstriction, predisposing patients to ischemia. The high frequency of stroke close to delivery and postpartum is also explained by preeclampsia/eclampsia. Epidemiologic studies show that both ischemic and hemorrhagic events in the first and second trimesters are minimal, but their frequency increases in the third trimester and closer to delivery, during delivery, and postpartum.[3,7–10]

Endocrine and Hematological Changes

Estrogen and progesterone, the 2 main hormones during pregnancy, are at first secreted by the corpus luteum, and later by the placenta. The estrogen level begins to increase after 100 days, reaching maximum by the last month of pregnancy. The progesterone concentration in the body increases during the first 3 months of pregnancy and then more rapidly by the end of the pregnancy.[11]

Estrogen stimulates the production of clotting factors in the liver, leading to increase of procoagulants during pregnancy starting in the second and progressing to the third trimester. This increase explains why women in the third trimester are more prone to thrombotic complications. Recent systematic reviews showed that most inherited thrombophilias, including factor V Leiden mutation, prothrombin G20210A mutation, protein S deficiency, protein C deficiency, and antithrombin deficiency, were associated with a significant increase in the risk of pregnancy-related venous thrombosis and embolism.[12] Antiphospholipid antibody syndrome is an acquired procoagulant state in which thrombi often form in both arteries and veins. The resulting hypercoagulable state, in association with a venous stasis condition, may likely account for an increased risk of thromboembolic complications, in particular, during the third trimester and the puerperium.[7]

Body Water and Metabolic Changes

Another important alteration that occurs during pregnancy is an increased retention of water. The period of maximal water retention is associated with an increased elaboration of estrogens and adrenocorticoids, which usually increase almost 4-fold by the end of pregnancy. Estrogens also have a lipotrophic effect, which is partly responsible for changes that occur in total neutral fat, serum phospholipids, and circulating cholesterol during pregnancy. Steroid hormones also cause changes in carbohydrate metabolism, increasing the level of plasma glucose.[11] These changes increase the risk of hypertension, hyperlipidemia, and glucose intolerance during pregnancy, which increases the risk of cerebrovascular complications.

Cardiovascular Changes

Cardiac output increases 30% to 50% during the course of pregnancy because of plasma volume expansion and estrogen-mediated increase in heart rate. Progesterone levels increase toward the end of the pregnancy and act to increase venous distensibility. This low-resistance state allows the vasculature to accommodate higher volumes while maintaining pressures consistent with the nonpregnant state under regular circumstances, but, along with compromised venous return from the inferior vena cava, it results in dependent edema, varicose veins, hemorrhoids, labial varicosities, and an increased risk of venous thromboembolism.[7,13]

PREGNANCY-SPECIFIC CAUSES OF STROKE
Preeclampsia and Eclampsia

Preeclampsia and eclampsia are the most pregnancy-specific causes of stroke. Preeclampsia/eclampsia usually develop in the third trimester or within 48 hours after delivery. Delayed preeclampsia and eclampsia may occur beyond 48 hours of delivery and up to 4 weeks postpartum. Preeclampsia is a syndrome unique to human pregnancy and the puerperium characterized by the new onset of hypertension

(>140/90 mm Hg) and proteinuria after 20 weeks of gestation in previously normotensive and normoproteinuric women. In eclampsia, patients have the same findings as in preeclampsia, with the addition of generalized seizures. In the United States, preeclampsia/eclampsia affects 5% to 8% of all pregnant women and is the third leading cause of maternal mortality.[14,15] It is more common in African American and Hispanic women than in white women and in those who are aged more than 35 years, have a history of hypertension, diabetes, connective tissue disorders, multiple pregnancies, body mass index more than 35, and family history of preeclampsia.

In preeclampsia/eclampsia, vascular mediators are released that injure vascular endothelia and provoke vasoconstriction. In addition, preeclampsia/eclampsia is associated with an increase of soluble FMS-like tyrosine kinase by hypoxic trophoblasts, which bind placental and vascular endothelial growth factors. Decrease in those factors may be associated with endothelial injury and lead to cerebral infarction or hemorrhage. Some autoptic findings in patients with hemorrhage caused by eclampsia are similar to those found in patients with hypertensive encephalopathy and are attributable to the abrupt increase in blood pressure, vasodilatation, and leakage from injured capillary and arteriolar endothelia.[7] A common complication of eclampsia is the reversible posterior leukoencephalopathy syndrome. The clinical findings are characterized by agitation and restlessness, confusion, seizures, and visual dysfunction that includes visual hallucinations and cortical blindness. Brain imaging shows white matter hyperintensities maximal in the occipital and posterior temporal white matter but sparing the paramedian occipital striate regions. This syndrome is likely a capillary leak syndrome related to endothelial dysfunction and increased body fluid volumes. Irreversible tissue damage develops if the blood pressure increases and edema are not treated rapidly and effectively.[16] Neuroimaging is the most reliable tool for evaluation of the neurologic complications of preeclampsia/eclampsia. MRI abnormalities in preeclampsia are usually present in the white matter only, whereas, in eclampsia, patients often show a characteristic curvilinear abnormality at the gray-white matter junction and predominantly in the frontal and parietal areas. Because of their small size, microhemorrhages or microinfarcts may not be seen even on high-resolution MRI; thus, vasogenic edema is the most common abnormality observed.[7,16] Management of patients with preeclampsia/eclampsia is lowering of blood pressure, decreasing brain edema, treatment of seizures, and delivery of the baby. Low-dose aspirin may reduce the occurrence of preeclampsia and its associated complications.[7] Prevention of eclampsia-related strokes and hemorrhages should be directed toward aggressive treatment of preeclampsia with control of hypertension.

Reversible Cerebral Vasoconstriction Syndrome

The reversible cerebral vasoconstriction syndrome (RCVS) is another important cause of stroke in pregnant and puerperal women, originally described as postpartum angiopathy. It applies to a group of disorders with different causes, but similar clinical, laboratory, imaging, and angiographic features characterized by prolonged, but reversible, changes in medium-sized and large-sized cerebral arteries.[7] Patients present clinically with the acute onset of severe recurrent headaches and angiographic evidence of segmental narrowing or beading of intracranial arteries. The headache often begins abruptly and has been called thunderclap headache. The vasoconstriction may persist for days and weeks and can progress to brain infarctions and subarachnoid and brain hemorrhages. Patients may, rarely, develop a fulminant course with poor outcome and death.[7,8]

The cause of RCVS is still not completely understood. Some substances associated with RCVS include selective serotonin reuptake inhibitors, phenylpropanolamine, cocaine, amphetamines, triptans, and cannabis. Women with a history of migraine are more susceptible to RCVS. The frequent occurrence of RCVS during the post-partum period is possibly caused by rapid decrease of progesterone, which acts as a vasodilator. Patients with RCVS who are untreated may develop the reversible posterior leukoencephalopathy syndrome.

Diagnosis of RCVS depends on showing vasoconstriction in the cerebral vessels. Digital subtraction angiography and CT angiography are useful diagnostic tools, but radiation and use of contrast limit their use in pregnancy. Magnetic resonance angiography has low sensitivity for RCVS. Neuroimaging, even MRI, has limited potential early in the course; in up to one-third of RCVS cases, brain images are normal. Angiographic findings are also not specific for RCVS and can be seen in any cerebral vasculitis. Transcranial Doppler can show increased velocities early, in the absence of focal neurologic symptoms.[7] Hemorrhages may be seen in up to one-third of patients with RCVS; they can be multifocal and can coexist with ischemic strokes. The mechanisms of hemorrhages in RCVS are most likely reperfusion of brain ischemic lesions and acute hypertension. Management of RCVS is mostly based on experience because no clinical trial results are available. Sidorov and colleagues[7] favor management of hypertension and prescription of calcium-channel blockers.[7,16] Long-acting verapamil in doses of 180 to 360 mg daily has, in their experience, almost always been effective if introduced early in the course.[7] Nonsteroidal antiinflammatory agents can be used to treat the headache; the blood pressure, if high, should be lowered to normal.

CEREBRAL VENOUS AND SINUS THROMBOSIS

Cerebral venous and sinus thrombosis (CVST) is another common cause of stroke in pregnancy and the puerperium. In a large US population-based study, the incidence of CVST in pregnancy and the puerperium was estimated at 11.6 cases per 100,000 deliveries; the incidence in developing countries is higher at 4.5 per 1000 obstetric cases. Water restriction, multiparity, anemia, vegetarian diet, and increased homocysteine levels explain the high incidence of CVST in these countries.[3] Although preeclampsia/eclampsia and RCVS are conditions primarily affecting arteries, arterioles, and capillaries, the pathophysiology of CVST concerns abnormal venous drainage and increase in intracranial pressures related to venous obstruction. Another important pathophysiologic factor is hypercoagulability toward the end of pregnancy caused by the increase of procoagulants and suppression of factors inhibiting coagulation, such as protein S and protein C. Several studies report a higher frequency of postpartum than antepartum CVST and venous strokes.[3,10] This may, at least in part, be related to the method of delivery. Cesarean section seems to be associated with a higher rate of CVST, simply because any surgery is associated with higher frequency of venous thrombosis. Another explanation is reduction of protein C level after surgery, which in turn activates protein C.[17] In addition, infection, which is more common postpartum, has been established as a risk factor for puerperium CVST. Blood loss during delivery may result in dehydration and predispose to the formation of thrombi.[7]

The clinical presentation of CVST in pregnancy and the puerperium is not different from that in nonpregnant women. The major clinical features include headache, altered consciousness, and focal neurologic signs, as well as seizures. Headache caused by increasing intracranial pressure is the earliest, and sometimes the only, symptom. Clinical presentation and prognosis depend on the presence, location, and extent of any brain lesion and the number and location of dural sinuses involved.

The sagittal and lateral sinuses are most often involved. Patients with exclusive involvement of deep draining veins may present with no other signs but encephalopathy, which may be misleading and delay diagnosis.

For diagnosis of CVST, MRI and magnetic resonance venogram are the most reliable tools. Thrombi during the acute period image as an isointense signal on T1-weighted images and are hypointense in T2-weighted images; on T2*-weighted images, thrombi are often black. The MRI changes are best seen in the superior sagittal, lateral, and straight sinuses, and are often less obvious in cortical veins.

First choice in the acute treatment of CVST is anticoagulation with heparin or heparin analogs,[18] later followed by warfarin for 3 to 6 months unless a coagulopathy is discovered on evaluation, in which case the anticoagulation is continued. Because dabigatran and newer factor Xa inhibitors work quickly, they may replace heparin and warfarin as standard anticoagulant treatment, but there are restrictions for treatment in pregnancy.

OTHER CAUSES OF STROKE IN PREGNANCY
Choriocarcinoma

Choriocarcinoma is a malignant neoplasm that arises from placental trophoblastic tissue, usually following a molar pregnancy but also term delivery, abortion, or ectopic pregnancy. The incidence of choriocarcinoma is 1 per 50,000 full-term pregnancies, but 1 per 30 molar pregnancies. Its role in stroke is related to the strong tendency of choriocarcinoma to metastasize to the brain, which can happen in up to 25% of patients.[19,20] Trophoblasts can invade brain vessels, just as they do in the uterus. Cerebral ischemia may be the result of thrombotic process in damaged vessels or a consequence of trophoblastic cerebrovascular embolism. Other vessels may be eroded, with development of aneurysms or bleeding into the tumor mass or surrounding space. Hemorrhage into choriocarcinoma brain metastases and into infarcts is characteristic of choriocarcinomas.[7,8] The clinical presentation of cerebral involvement includes headache, focal neurologic deficits, seizures, encephalopathy, signs of increased intracranial pressure, and excessively increased β human choriogonadotrophic hormone level.[21]

Peripartum Cardiomyopathy

Peripartum cardiomyopathy is a rare dilating cardiomyopathy that develops in the last gestational month of pregnancy or in the first 5 months after delivery. It occurs in the absence of any preexisting heart disease and is most common in older, black, and multiparous women. The incidence of systemic embolism is estimated at approximately 25% to 40%; however, ischemic strokes are seen in only 5% of patients. The diagnosis is made by exclusion, based on the clinical presentation and echocardiographic findings. Management is the same as in other types of dilated cardiomyopathy.[7,21]

Amniotic Fluid Embolism

Amniotic fluid embolism (AFE) is another rare complication of pregnancy that potentially can lead to stroke. The incidence is estimated at approximately 1 in 13,000 to 56,000 deliveries. The risk factors for AFE are maternal age more than 35 years, cesarean section, forceps-assisted or vacuum-assisted delivery, placenta previa, placental abruption, eclampsia, and fetal distress. AFE occurs in a setting of a disrupted barrier between the amniotic fluid and the maternal circulation. The clinical presentation is characterized by systemic hypotension, cardiac dysrhythmia, cyanosis, dyspnea, and even respiratory arrest, pulmonary edema, and altered level of consciousness. Seizures occur at presentation in 10% to 20% of patients. The true incidence of ischemic brain infarcts in AFE is unknown. The mechanism includes paradoxic embolism and severe vascular collapse.[7,16]

Paradoxic Embolism

The risk of deep venous thrombosis in the legs and pelvis increases during pregnancy and the postpartum period. Although it is unknown whether paradoxic emboli through a patent foramen ovale also occur more frequently, it is reasonable to have a high clinical suspicion for this potential cause.

GENERAL CAUSES OF STROKE IN YOUNG WOMEN

Other causes of stroke in pregnancy are those that also occur in nonpregnant young women. They include carotid and vertebral artery dissection, cardiac arrhythmias, heart valve disease, cerebral vasculitis, arteriovenous malformations, migraine, moyamoya disease, and sickle cell anemia. Carotid and vertebral artery dissection are more common during delivery owing to the increase in blood pressure or hyperextension of the neck during general anesthesia. General vascular risk factors like hypertension, diabetes, and hyperlipidemia play an increasing role in the cause of stroke during pregnancy and puerperium because of the increasing occurrence of obesity and increasing maternal age.

SAFETY OF BRAIN IMAGING DURING PREGNANCY

MRI and CT are the 2 major imaging technologies used in the diagnosis of stroke, but several concerns about fetal exposure to radiation or magnetic field arise for the clinician.

CT

Evaluation with CT involves exposure to ionizing radiation, and the harmful effects depend on the stage of gestation at which the fetus is exposed and the total dose of radiation absorbed. Fetal exposure to ionizing radiation from CT of the maternal head is extremely low. Potential risk of birth defects caused by radiation are limited to the embryogenesis period in the first few weeks. According to guidelines for diagnostic imaging during pregnancy, radiation exposure less than 5 rad has not been associated with an increase in fetal anomalies or pregnancy loss. CT scan of the head gives a fetal exposure of less than 1 rad and so can be safely performed in pregnant women, especially if hemorrhage is suspected. The development of various cancers in childhood is another concern for ionizing radiation in utero. It was estimated that 1 in 2000 children exposed to ionizing radiation develop leukemia, compared with a background rate of 1 in 3000. Thus, the risk of carcinogenesis may be higher, but was estimated not to exceed 1 in 1000 children per 1 rad.[22] Iodine contrast medium given to the mother crosses the placental barrier and has the potential to depress fetal and neonatal thyroid function, so a CT perfusion study should therefore be avoided. Neonatal thyroid function should be checked during the first week if iodinated contrast has been given during pregnancy.

MRI

MRI uses hydrogen proton energy and is a safer and more useful tool for evaluation of stroke ischemia during pregnancy. Although there have been no documented adverse fetal effects reported, the National Radiologic Protection Board arbitrarily advises against the use of MRI during the first trimester. More recent data suggest that MRI is safe in any trimester of pregnancy.[23] All available safety data are for 1.5-T MRI. MRI safety in pregnancy for 3-T system remains unknown.[24] Even though noncontrast MRI is used to diagnose stroke, gadolinium-based contrast (GBC) studies may be useful for neck MR angiograms. At this stage, there is no agreement on the safety of the use of GBC in pregnancy. Animal models have shown growth retardation as a result of administration of GBC; however, no controlled human studies have confirmed these findings.[7] As a result, GBC is considered as a category C substance for use in pregnancy. This category includes substances for which there is evidence supporting adverse effects in the fetus from animal models.

STROKE PREVENTION DURING PREGNANCY
Antiplatelet and Anticoagulant Therapy

Minimal data exist on preventive treatment of stroke in pregnancy, and there are no randomized controlled trials.[7,8,16,25] Use of aspirin, in particular, has been a source of debate because animal studies have suggested an increased risk of congenital abnormalities. In addition, several human studies reported increased risks of specific malformations including heart defects, neural tube defects, hypospadias, cleft palate, gastroschisis, and pyloric stenosis.[26] However, a subsequent meta-analysis in 2003 failed to find any increased risk associated with aspirin, including placental abruption, fetal intraventricular hemorrhage, or congenital malformations.[27] A recent meta-analysis suggests that aspirin is beneficial in preventing preeclampsia when started earlier than 16 weeks' gestation, but not when initiated after 16 weeks. In that study, early treatment with aspirin also resulted in a decrease in gestational hypertension and preterm birth.[28]

Owing to the limited data and lack of randomized controlled trials, current guidelines regarding the recommendations of aspirin in pregnant women vary. According to the American Heart Association/American Stroke Association guidelines, women at increased risk of stroke in whom antiplatelet therapy would likely be considered outside of pregnancy may be considered for unfractionated heparin (UFH) or low-molecular-weight heparin (LMWH) during the first trimester, followed by low-dose aspirin.[29] The American College of Chest Physicians has published guidelines for the management of thromboembolism and thrombophilia in pregnancy, and, although they do not specifically address stroke, they recommend low-dose aspirin throughout pregnancy for women at high risk of preeclampsia.[30] This may include women with preexisting hypertension, diabetes, renal disease, obesity, age greater than 35 years, and prior eclampsia.

In conclusion, antiplatelet therapy with low-dose aspirin (<150 mg) is considered safe during the second and the third trimesters of pregnancy, but the risk for its use during the first trimester is unknown. There are virtually no data available regarding use of other antiplatelet agents, such as clopidogrel or aspirin-dipyridamole, in pregnancy.

The American Heart Association/American Stroke Association considers 3 prevention options for pregnant women with ischemic stroke and high-risk thromboembolic conditions such as hypercoagulable state or mechanical heart valves:

- UFH throughout pregnancy
- LMWH throughout pregnancy
- UFH/LMWH until week 13, followed by warfarin until the middle of the third trimester, then UFH/LMWH up to the time of delivery.[29]

The American College of Chest Physicians has identical recommendations for high-risk women with mechanical valves.[29,30]

Women with a history of venous thromboembolism plus a known thrombophilia, particularly antithrombin III deficiency, antiphospholipid antibody syndrome, prothrombin gene mutation, or factor V Leiden, may be treated with prophylactic LMWH or UFH during pregnancy followed by postpartum anticoagulation with warfarin.[8] For women with antiphospholipid antibody syndrome and no history of venous thromboembolism, but recurrent pregnancy loss, prophylactic UFH or LMWH plus aspirin throughout pregnancy is recommended.[8,29,30] LMWH is the most attractive option owing to more predictable dose response and ease of use compared with UFH, as well as decreased risk of osteoporosis and thrombocytopenia.[8] Some investigators suggest a transition to UFH just before delivery to decrease the risk of epidural hematoma associated with regional anesthesia.[31] American Heart Association/American Stroke Association stroke secondary prevention guidelines recommend anticoagulation for at least 3 months in the setting of CVST, followed by antiplatelet therapy.[29]

In conclusion, anticoagulation therapy during pregnancy continues to be a controversial topic. The lack of systematic studies on the use of anticoagulation therapy during pregnancy makes it difficult to provide guidelines. Agents that can, in general, be used for anticoagulation include heparin, LMWH, warfarin, direct thrombin inhibitors (hirudin, argatroban and dabigatran), and factor Xa inhibitors (apixaban and rivaroxaban). Warfarin is known to cross the placental barrier and cause teratogenic side effects. It has been associated with 14.6% to 56% risk of miscarriage and 30% risk of congenital anomalies if used from week 4 to week 8. It may cause bleeding if used later in pregnancy. Neither heparin nor LMWH cross the placental barrier, and both are considered safe in pregnancy. The potential complications include hemorrhage, reduced bone density, and heparin-induced thrombocytopenia. LMWH has the advantage of a more stable coagulant response to fixed doses given twice daily, and has a lower incidence of thrombocytopenia and osteoporosis. Use of LMWH in pregnant women with mechanical valves has been controversial, owing to reports of maternal and fetal death. Overall, anticoagulation with warfarin is safe after the first trimester; before that, heparin or LMWH can be used. No data regarding the safety of dabigatran or factor Xa inhibitors in pregnancy are available,[7] but dabigatran is currently US Food and Drug Administration category C for pregnant women.

TREATMENT OF ACUTE PREGNANCY-RELATED STROKE

Treatment of acute arterial stroke in pregnancy is also controversial.

Thrombolytic Therapy

Early thrombolysis with intravenous tissue plasminogen activator (tPA) or mechanical clot removal are effective for acute ischemic arterial stroke.[32,33] There is no direct evidence for the safety of thrombolytic therapy in pregnancy, because pregnant women were excluded from randomized therapeutic trials. Several case reports of successful intravenous and intra-arterial tPA use during pregnancy in patients with stroke, pulmonary embolism and renal artery thrombosis were published recently with major improvement or complete resolution of neurologic function.[7,34] Even though, in many patients, it was safe with no complications, 1 review of 172 pregnant patients reported maternal hemorrhages in as many as 8%.[35] Another study revealed intracranial hemorrhage in 1 out of 11 pregnant women after off-label tPA use.[36] Teratogenicity has not been reported as a complication of thrombolytic therapy but too few cases have been treated during pregnancy to give general advice on tPA treatment during pregnancy.

Treatment of Hemorrhages in Pregnancy

There are no clear guidelines for medical treatment of subarachnoid or intracranial hemorrhage in pregnancy. Drugs like mannitol for increased intracranial pressure or nimodipine for vasospasm must be used with caution. Mannitol may result in fetal hypoxia and acid-base shifts, and nimodipine has been linked with teratogenicity in some animal studies.[8] However, in critically ill pregnant patients, the use of these agents, including potentially teratogenic anticonvulsants in case of seizures, may outweigh the risks. The decision to operate after intracerebal hemorrhage during pregnancy should be based on neurosurgical principles, and the method of delivery should be based on obstetric considerations. Historically, cesarean delivery has been advocated for women with intracranial hemorrhage, particularly recent subarachnoid hemorrhage, untreated ruptured arteriovenous malformations, or unclipped aneurysms, to avoid potential risks during labor and delivery. However, studies suggest that outcomes of vaginal and cesarean delivery are probably equivalent after intracranial hemorrhage.[25,37] However, cesarean delivery may be a risk factor for postpartum stroke caused by cerebral venous thrombosis.

SUMMARY

Ischemic infarcts and hemorrhages in pregnancy are uncommon, but there is an approximately 2.4-times higher stroke risk for pregnant women, including the initial 6 weeks postpartum, compared with nonpregnant young women. Most strokes are seen in the third trimester and postpartum and the cause is most often related to one of the following 3 conditions: preeclampsia/eclampsia, RCVS, and CVST. Rarer causes include choriocarcinoma, peripartum cardiomyopathy, and AFE. All other known causes of stroke, seen in nonpregnant women, can also be relevant during pregnancy, including hypertension, diabetes, vasculitis, dissection, arteriovenous malformations, or aneurysms.

Women at the highest risk for pregnancy-related stroke are those who are more than 35 years of age; those who are of African American ethnicity; and those with preeclampsia/eclampsia/gestational hypertension, thrombophilias, migraine headaches, diabetes, prepregnancy hypertension, hyperemesis gravidarum, anemia, thrombocytopenia, postpartum hemorrhage, fluid and electrolyte disorders, and infections. The clinical and therapeutic approach to women with stroke during pregnancy should be similar to the approach to stroke in young adults. MRI and magnetic resonance venogram are generally considered the gold standard for the diagnosis of ischemic stroke and cerebral venous thrombosis, respectively. Timing of scans may depend on the stage of pregnancy and the risk/benefit ratio of performing these scans. The risk from MRI is generally considered lower after the first trimester, and the risk with administration of gadolinium is still being debated.

Strategies for stroke prevention should take into account the competing risks to mother and fetus. Treatment of acute stroke in pregnant women is still controversial, but not strictly contraindicated. Several case reports have documented successful reperfusion, in addition to satisfactory maternal and fetal outcomes. Aspirin and warfarin are safe in the second and third trimesters. However, there are no trials of anticoagulation or antiplatelet therapies of stroke prevention in pregnancy.

REFERENCES

1. Kittner SJ, Stern BJ, Feeser BR, et al. Pregnancy and the risk of stroke. N Engl J Med 1996;335:768–74.

2. Liang CC, Chang SD, Lai SL, et al. Stroke complicating pregnancy and the puerperium. Eur J Neurol 2006;13(11):1256–60.
3. Lanska DJ, Kryscio RJ. Risk factors for peripartum and postpartum stroke and intracranial venous thrombosis. Stroke 2000;31:1274–82.
4. Kuklina EV, Tong X, Bansil P, et al. Trends in pregnancy hospitalizations that included a stroke in the United States from 1994 to 2007: reasons for concern? Stroke 2011;42(9):2564–70.
5. Zhang X, Shu XO, Gao YT, et al. Pregnancy, childrearing, and risk of stroke in Chinese women. Stroke 2009;40(8):2680–4.
6. Skilton MR, Bonnet F, Begg LM, et al. Childbearing, child-rearing, cardiovascular risk factors, and progression of carotid intima-media thickness: the Cardiovascular Risk in Young Finns study. Stroke 2010;41(7):1332–7.
7. Sidorov EV, Feng WF, Caplan LR. Stroke in pregnant and postpartum women. Expert Rev Cardiovasc Ther 2011;9:1235–47.
8. Tate J, Bushnell C. Pregnancy and stroke risk in women. Womens Health 2011;7: 363–74.
9. Jeng JS, Tang SC, Yip PK. Incidence and etiologies of stroke during pregnancy and puerperium as evidenced in Taiwanese women. Cerebrovasc Dis 2004;18:290–5.
10. Jaigobin C, Silver FL. Stroke and pregnancy. Stroke 2000;31:2948–51.
11. Feldt-Rasmussen U, Mathiesen ER. Endocrine disorders in pregnancy: physiological and hormonal aspects of pregnancy. Best Pract Res Clin Endocrinol Metab 2011;25:875–84.
12. Gerhardt A, Scharf AE, Beckmann MW, et al. Prothrombin and factor V mutations in women with a history of thrombosis during pregnancy and the puerperium. N Engl J Med 2000;342:374–80.
13. Clark SL, Cotoon DB, Lee W, et al. Central hemodynamic assessment of normal term pregnancy. Am J Obstet Gynecol 1989;161:1439–42.
14. Turner JA. Diagnosis and management of preeclampsia: an update. Int J Womens Health 2010;2:327–37.
15. Morales-Vidal S, Schneck MJ, Flaster MS, et al. Stroke- and pregnancy-induced hypertensive syndromes. Women Health 2011;7:283–92.
16. Dirge MV, Caplan LR. Uncommon causes of stroke. Cambridge (UK): Cambridge University Press; 2008.
17. Andersson TR, Berner NS, Larsen ML, et al. Plasma heparin cofactor II, protein C and antithrombin in elective surgery. Acta Chir Scand 1987;153:291–6.
18. Cheng SJ, Chen PH, Chen LA, et al. Stroke during pregnancy and puerperium: clinical perspectives. Taiwan J Obstet Gynecol 2010;49:395–400.
19. Ilancheran A, Ratnam SS, Baratham G. Metastatic cerebral choriocarcinoma with primary neurological presentation. Gynecol Oncol 1988;29:361–4.
20. Huang CY, Chen CA, Hsieh CY, et al. Intracerebral hemorrhage as initial presentation of gestational choriocarcinoma: a case report and literature review. Int J Gynecol Cancer 2007;17:1166–71.
21. Del Zotto E, Giossi A, Volonghi I, et al. Ischemic stroke during pregnancy and puerperium. Stroke Res Treat 2011;606780 (published online).
22. Guidelines for diagnostic imaging during pregnancy. The American College of Obstetricians and Gynecologists. Int J Gynecol Obstet 1995;51:288–91.
23. Shellock FG, Crues JV. MR procedures: biologic effects, safety, and patient care. Radiology 2004;232:635–52.
24. Levine D. Obstetric MRI. J Magn Reson Imaging 2006;24:1–15.
25. Pathan M, Kittner SJ. Pregnancy and stroke. Curr Neurol Neurosci Rep 2003;3(1): 27–31.

26. Kozer E, Nikfar S, Costei A, et al. Aspirin consumption during the first trimester of pregnancy and congenital anomalies: a meta-analysis. Am J Obstet Gynecol 2002;187:1623–30.
27. Coomarasamy A, Honest H, Papaioannou S, et al. Aspirin for prevention of preeclampsia in women with historical risk factors: a systematic review. Obstet Gynecol 2003;101:1319–32.
28. Bujold E, Roberge S, Lacasse Y, et al. Prevention of preeclampsia and intra-uterine growth restriction with aspirin started in early pregnancy. Obstet Gynecol 2010;116:402–14.
29. Furie K, Kasner S, Adams R, et al. Guidelines for the prevention of stroke in patients with stroke or transient ischemic attack. A guideline for healthcare professionals from the American Heart Association/American Stroke Association. Stroke 2011;42:227–76.
30. Bates S, Greer I, Pabinger I, et al. Venous thromboembolism, thrombophilia, antithrombotic therapy, and pregnancy. Chest 2008;133:844S–86S.
31. Cronin C, Weisman C, Llinas R. Stroke treatment: beyond the three hour window and in the pregnant patient. Ann N Y Acad Sci 2008;1142:159–78.
32. Davis S, Donnan G. The ECASS III results and the tPA paradox. Int J Stroke 2009; 4:17–8.
33. Smith WS, Sung G, Saver J, et al. Mechanical thrombectomy for acute ischemic stroke: final results of the multi MERCI trial. Stroke 2008;39:1205–12.
34. Murugappan A, Coplin W, Al-Sadat A, et al. Thrombolytic therapy of acute ischemic stroke during pregnancy. Neurology 2006;66:768–70.
35. Turrentine MA, Braems G, Ramirez MM. Use of thrombolytics for the treatment of thromboembolic disease during pregnancy. Obstet Gynecol Surv 1995;50: 534–41.
36. Aleu A, Mellado P, Lichy C, et al. Hemorrhagic complications after off-label thrombolysis for ischemic stroke. Stroke 2007;38:417–22.
37. Treadwill S, Thanvi B, Robinson T. Stroke in pregnancy and the puerperium. Postgrad Med J 2008;84:238–45.

Sleep Disorders in Pregnancy
Implications, Evaluation, and Treatment

Sally Ibrahim, MD[a],*, Nancy Foldvary-Schaefer, DO, MS[b]

KEYWORDS

- Pregnancy • Sleep • Restless legs syndrome • Insomnia • Obstructive sleep apnea
- Maternal-fetal health

KEY POINTS

- Sleep problems in pregnancy are common and may affect pregnancy.
- Restless legs syndrome is very common during pregnancy and is easily diagnosed with 4 clinical criteria.
- Shorter sleep duration in pregnancy is associated with increased morbidity, such as gestational diabetes and preeclampsia.
- Snoring and obstructive sleep apnea (OSA) are associated with increased risk of gestational diabetes, preeclampsia, and pregnancy-induced hypertension.

Sleep complaints are commonly reported during pregnancy. The dynamic physiologic and physical changes across pregnancy affect sleep and wakefulness producing sleep disturbances, which causes sleep disorders in some cases. Up to one-third or more of pregnant women report some type of sleep problem.[1] Although sleep disorders are prevalent, sleep complaints are seldom discussed, and most women do not receive information about sleep in pregnancy.[2] Moreover, sleep disorders may have implications on maternal-fetal health. This review illustrates common sleep disorders in pregnancy and emphasizes the health outcomes and potential therapies.

SLEEP DURATION, ARCHITECTURE, AND QUALITY

Sleep in pregnancy is described objectively and subjectively. Sleep duration dynamically changes across pregnancy. Sleep duration increases in the first trimester and returns closer to prepartum values by the second trimester, which then subsequently decreases until its minimum postpartum value.[3] Subjective sleep quality also declines

Dr Ibrahim has nothing to disclose. Dr Foldvary-Schaefer receives research support from CleveMed and Teva Neurosciences. He is a paid speaker for Jazz Pharmaceuticals.
a Cleveland Clinic Sleep Disorders Center, Neurological Institute, 9500 Euclid Avenue, FA 20, Cleveland, OH 44195, USA; b Cleveland Clinic Lerner College of Medicine, Cleveland Clinic Sleep Disorders Center, 9500 Euclid Avenue, FA 20, Cleveland, OH 44195, USA
* Corresponding author.
E-mail address: Ibrahis2@ccf.org

across pregnancy, starting in the first trimester.[1,4] Nocturnal awakenings, reported by up to 72% of pregnant women,[2] may play some role[3,4] and disturb sleep maintenance. Nocturia is reported, followed by other causes including frightened dreams, leg cramps, gastrointestinal problems (eg, reflux), discomfort (eg, backache), and, uncommonly, fetal movements.[2,3] Difficulty in returning to sleep after awakenings is especially problematic in the final trimester.[3] Polysomnographic (PSG) studies demonstrate objective changes in sleep architecture. Pregnancy affects sleep efficiency and wake after sleep onset (WASO). Sleep efficiency, defined as a percentage of time asleep/time in bed, may decrease in some patients. Decreased sleep efficiency is attributed to increased WASO and cortical arousals.[3]

Epidemiologic evidence indicates that short sleep duration is a risk factor for obesity and increased weight gain, glucose intolerance, hypertension (HTN), coronary artery disease (CAD), and other adverse conditions.[1] During pregnancy, similar adverse effects are recognized. Short sleep duration (≤ 5 hours) is associated with higher blood pressure in third trimester and risk of preeclampsia.[5] Less than 7 hours of sleep is associated with increased incidence of gestational diabetes mellitus (GDM) (odds ratio [OR] 11.7).[6] Environmental, social, and medical factors affect sleep duration and quality including African American race and higher body mass index (BMI, calculated as the weight in kilograms divided by height in meters squared).[1,5] Sleep disorders during pregnancy also affect sleep duration and quality, which are discussed subsequently.

INSOMNIA

Insomnia is defined as[7]

- A complaint or difficulty in initiating or maintaining sleep, or waking up too early or sleep that is chronically nonrestorative or poor in quality
- A difficulty that occurs despite the adequate opportunity and circumstances for sleep
- An association with some form of daytime impairment (fatigue, low energy, mood disturbance, excessive concern or worry about sleep, decline in school, work, social performance, or other symptom of sleep loss).

Insomnia is common in pregnancy. Longitudinal evaluation using the Women's Health Initiative Insomnia Rating Scale, found significant increases in insomnia from early pregnancy (38%) to late pregnancy (54%).[1] There are several types of insomnia. Insomnia may be directly related to pregnancy because of the adjustments to physical, hormonal, and metabolic changes. Insomnia may also coexist with psychiatric conditions, such as anxiety. Sleep initiation difficulties are a significant predictor of depression and anxiety in pregnancy.[8] Circadian factors may play some role in sleep initiation and maintenance. The normal diurnal circadian rhythm of melatonin secretion (increase during the dark-night period) is maintained during pregnancy. However, the nocturnal increase in melatonin amplitude increases with advancing pregnancy.[9] Abnormal melatonin secretion can alter sleep and is associated with adverse conditions, such as preeclampsia and spontaneous abortion.[9] Circadian rhythm disorders in pregnancy, however, have not been studied, and there are no evidenced-based uses for exogenous melatonin in pregnancy.

Insomnia management includes medications (**Table 1**) and nonpharmacologic therapies (**Table 2**). Drug therapy with sleep aids is seldom prescribed during pregnancy because of the concerns regarding adverse effects. Nonpharmacologic therapies for insomnia include improvement in sleep hygiene, relaxation, cognitive behavioral therapy, and other complimentary therapies.[10] Mindful yoga group interventions

---

Case Study

Clinical description: SN, a 30-year-old chef, was 13 weeks' pregnant with her second child. Her previous pregnancy 2 years ago was complicated by pregnancy-induced hypertension. After her first pregnancy, her blood pressure (BP) level returned to normal. With her current pregnancy, the BP had been in the high-normal range. SN was concerned about the recurrence of elevated BP and complications with her current pregnancy. On review of symptoms, SN stated that she did not sleep well. Sleep quality was worse during pregnancy. She described snoring almost nightly with multiple nocturnal awakenings. SN started snoring in adulthood after a 20-pound weight gain. Her husband noticed an increase in snoring during her pregnancies. SN was often so fatigued and tired during the day regardless of the amount of sleep she obtained the night before. Even with naps, she woke unrefreshed.

Discussion/analysis: SN is likely to have obstructive sleep apnea (OSA), worsening during pregnancy. OSA is associated with elevated BP and conditions such as preeclampsia and pregnancy-induced hypertension. Thus, SN possibly had OSA during her previous pregnancy. Because of the concerns of increasing BP levels in the current pregnancy, polysomnography was recommended, which revealed a moderate degree of OSA. She was subsequently treated with continuous positive airway pressure, which was tolerated well. SN reported having more refreshing sleep, nearly resolved nocturnal awakenings, and no longer had sleepiness during the day. Her husband was especially happy to have a quiet night without snoring. During the latter part of pregnancy, SN had high-normal BP readings but neither developed pregnancy-induced hypertension nor preeclampsia.

---

improved sleep in pregnancy measured by 72-hour actigraphy and self-report.[11] Exclusion of other emerging sleep disorders during pregnancy that effect sleep initiation and maintenance should be explored.

RESLTESS LEGS SYNDROME

Restless Legs Syndrome (RLS) is defined by the following 4 clinical criteria[7]:

- The patient reports an urge to move the legs, usually accompanied or caused by uncomfortable and unpleasant sensations in the legs.
- The urge to move or the unpleasant sensations start or worsen during periods of rest or inactivity, such as lying or sitting.
- The urge to move or the unpleasant sensations are partially or totally relieved by movement, such as walking or stretching, at least as long as the activity continues.
- The urge to move or the unpleasant sensations worsen, or only occur, in the evening or night.
- The condition is not better explained by another current sleep disorder, medical or neurologic disorder, mental disorder, medication use or substance-use disorder.

RLS is the most extensively studied sleep disorder in pregnancy. RLS may be primary/idiopathic or secondary to a medical condition. Primary RLS occurs sporadically or by autosomal dominant inheritance. Secondary causes of RLS include pregnancy, iron deficiency, uremia, peripheral neuropathy, and medications (eg, antihistamines, antidepressants, and dopamine antagonists). RLS should be differentiated from other conditions, such as nocturnal leg cramps, arthritic pain, positional discomfort/paresthesias, and unconscious foot movements (eg, foot tapping). RLS is characterized by a compelling urge to move more often than in other conditions.[7]

Pregnancy is a risk factor for the emergence or worsening of RLS. The prevalence of RLS in pregnancy is 26% to 32%.[12,13] Prevalence rates vary depending on the regional differences and study methodology. In severe cases, the prevalence is

Table 1
Insomnia medications, Food and Drug Administration (FDA), and pregnancy classes

Drug Class	Drug Name (Propriety)	Dosage (mg)	FDA Labeled for Insomnia	Pregnancy Class	Comments
Benzodiazepine receptor agonists	Zolpidem tartrate (Ambien)	5–10	Yes	C	Neonatal respiratory depression in late pregnancy
	Zolpidem extended release (Ambien CR)	6.25–12.5			
	Zaleplon (Sonata)	5–20	Yes	C	Shortest acting in this class
	Eszopiclone (Lunesta)	1–3	Yes	C	Headaches, metallic after-taste
Melatonin receptor agonist	Ramelteon (Rozerem)	8	Yes	C	Low potential for dependency
Benzodiazepines	Lorazepam (Ativan)	0.5–2	No (Anxiety)	D	Teratogenic effects, floppy infant syndrome, neonatal withdrawal, potential dependence
	Estazolam (ProSom)	0.5–2	Yes	X	
	Flurazepam (Dalmane)		Yes	X	
	Temazepam (Restoril)	25–30	Yes	X	
	Triazolam (Halcion)		Yes	X	
Sedating antidepressants	Doxepin (Silenor)	3–6	Yes	C	Sleep initiation and maintenance benefits
	Amitriptyline (Elavil)	25–75	No (Depression)	C	Anticholinergic side effects limit use
	Trazodone (Desyrel)	25–150	No (Depression)	C	Lower doses are typically beneficial
Antihistamines	Diphenhydramine (Benadryl; ingredient in many OTC sleep aids)	25–50	—	B	Morning grogginess
Other	Magnesium sulfate	—	No (Intravenous form for eclampsia)	A/C - depends on producer	Daily requirements in pregnancy 360 mg elemental Mg

Food and Drug Administration designated safety classification: Pregnancy Categories A–D, X:
A: Adequate and controlled studies in pregnancy fail to demonstrate a risk to the fetus; possibility of fetal harm seems remote.
B: Animal studies have not demonstrated a fetal risk but no controlled studies in pregnant women, or animal studies show possible risk but controlled studies in women do not demonstrate risk.
C: Animal studies have revealed adverse effects on the fetus (teratogenic, embryocidal) and there are no adequate/controlled studies in women. Possible use despite potential risk only if the potential benefit justifies possible risk.
D: Evidence of human fetal risk. Use in pregnant women may be acceptable despite the risk, for example, the drug is needed in a life-threatening situation or for a serious disease when safer drugs cannot be used.
X: Evidence in animals or humans of fetal abnormalities or fetal risk. Risk of use clearly outweighs any possible benefit; drug is contraindicated.
Abbreviation: OTC, over the counter.

Table 2
Nonpharmacologic therapies and sleep hygiene for insomnia in pregnancy

Daytime Practices	Indication
Set consistent regular bed and wake times.	This will help maintain a sleep rhythm
Avoid long and late evening naps. If a nap is taken, it should be short (~20 min)	Naps steal sleep pressure away from the night sleep, making sleep initiation difficult
Address mood concerns (ie, anxiety, depression) and physical complaints, such as low back pain/discomfort	Depressive and anxiety disorders are common in insomnia. Pain and discomfort may alter usual sleeping position and limit comfortable sleep
Consider implementation of complimentary therapies, such as relaxation and mindful yoga	These may be helpful in reducing anxiety and stress and may promote sleep initiation
Night Time Practices at Bed Time	
Practice progressive muscle relaxation and perform other soothing behaviors	Relaxation promotes sleep, reduces tension, and quiets the mind to prepare for sleep
Avoid watching TV, electronic pads/computers, texting, and use of other electronics in the bed	Alerting activities along with light exposure diminish sleep initiation processes
Avoid stimulants such as caffeine, smoking, and alcohol within 6 h of bed time	Stimulants interfere with sleepiness and sleep onset. Alcohol interferes with sleep quality
In Bed and During the Sleep Period	
Use a comfortable bed and pillow support	To support the back as the abdomen enlarges
Use the bed only for sleep and sex	This helps promote positive sleep associations
Avoid thinking or worrying in bed. Avoid watching the clock or worrying about time	Mental activities, especially negative, can alter the body's ability to sleep
If one cannot sleep within 15–20 min, get out of bed. Do something calm and relaxing in a dim lighting until feeling sleepy again	This will help to reinstate the sleep state and help the body to associate the bed with sleep

15%.[12] Symptoms usually develop or increase with advancing pregnancy.[1,12] Using a validated RLS severity scale prospectively, the prevalence of severe RLS increased from 15% in the first trimester to nearly one third of patients in the third trimester.[1] Transient RLS resolves quickly postpartum within the first month but can recur with subsequent pregnancies.[12] Patients who had RLS before pregnancy typically return to baseline after delivery. Although RLS during pregnancy is prevalent, the disorder is frequently misdiagnosed or ignored by clinicians.[13] Nonetheless, RLS adversely affects maternal sleep duration, sleep quality, use of sleep aids, and daytime functioning.[12,13] RLS, especially when severe, is associated with increased cardiovascular disease, such as HTN, cerebrovascular disease, and CAD.[14]

The pathophysiology of RLS in pregnancy, as in the general population, involves iron along with dopaminergic neurons that modulate nociceptive pathways.[7] Because of the precipitous decline in RLS after delivery, hormonal and metabolic changes likely play a role. A prospective study examined these changes.[15] Pregnancy-related RLS was associated with a more pronounced physiologic elevation in estradiol levels compared with controls. The antidopaminergic effects of estrogen may account for increasing RLS toward the end of pregnancy when estrogen levels are the highest.

Although hemodilution and increased fetal demand imply a possible role for iron in RLS, many women have normal levels of iron and appropriate iron intake.[12,15]

Studies on therapeutic interventions of RLS during pregnancy are lacking. The major goal of therapy is to provide symptomatic relief (**Fig. 1**).[16] In mild cases, conservative measures are recommended. In moderate to severe cases, pharmacologic therapy may be recommended. Dopaminergic agents are the drugs of choice in RLS.[16] The non–ergo-derived dopamine agonists (eg, ropinirole and pramipexole) are approved for RLS, but pregnancy safety data are limited. Opioids are also efficacious. Side effects and possible neonatal withdrawal syndrome may limit use during pregnancy. Benzodiazepines may be effective, but teratogenic effects limit their usage. In a case report, intravenous magnesium sulfate used in preterm labor completely resolved RLS.[17] Magnesium has a depressing effect on neuronal excitability and may alleviate RLS.[17] Future studies are needed for RLS treatment in pregnancy.

SLEEP-DISORDERED BREATHING

OSA, the most common form of sleep-disordered breathing (SDB), is characterized by repetitive episodes of upper airway obstruction resulting in partial or complete airflow cessation, causing oxygen desaturations and arousals from sleep. Patients may report snoring, witnessed apneas, nocturnal awakenings, nocturia, unrefreshing sleep, as well as excessive daytime fatigue and sleepiness. The disorder is diagnosed by over-night PSG based on the apnea-hypopnea index (AHI: mild, 5–<15; moderate, 15–<30; severe, ≥30; **Box 1**).[7]

OSA may develop or worsen during pregnancy and affect maternal-fetal health. The prevalence of OSA in pregnancy is unknown because of the lack of epidemiologic studies that use objective testing. Many studies rely on subjective tools for diagnosis. Using the Berlin screening questionnaire, 25% of pregnant women are suspects for OSA.[18] Frequent snoring, the most common symptom of OSA, is reported in 16% during late pregnancy.[1] Snoring nearly doubles from prepregnancy to the final month of pregnancy along with other emerging symptoms, such as witnessed apneic episodes.[19] BMI and large neck girth are risk factors for symptom development as well as severity and worsening of OSA symptoms in pregnancy.[18,19] Although the risk of OSA is higher in patients who are obese, patients who are not obese can

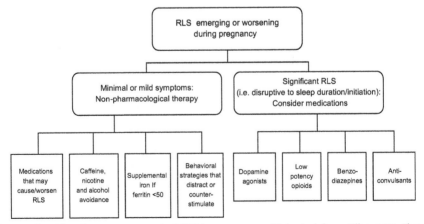

Fig. 1. Algorithm for management of RLS in pregnancy. (*Adapted from* Silber MH, Ehrenberg BL, Allen RP, et al. An algorithm for the management of restless legs syndrome. Mayo Clin Proc 2004;79(7):916–22; with permission.)

Box 1
Diagnostic criteria of OSA

Criteria: 1, 2, and 4 OR 3 and 4 satisfy the criteria

1. One of the following applies

   a. The patient complains of unintentional sleep episodes during wakefulness, daytime sleepiness, unrefreshing sleep, fatigue, or insomnia

   b. The patient wakes with holding his/her breath, gasping, or choking

   c. The bed partner reports loud snoring, breathing interruptions, or both during the patient's sleep

2. Polysomnographic recording shows

   a. Five or more scoreable respiratory events per hour of sleep (Scoreable respiratory events: apneas, hypopneas, or respiratory effort related arousals)

   b. Evidence of respiratory effort during all or a portion of each respiratory event

3. Polysomnographic recording shows

   a. Fifteen or more scoreable respiratory events per hour of sleep

   b. Evidence of respiratory effort during all or a portion of each respiratory event

4. The disorder is not better explained by another current sleep disorder, medical or neurologic disorder, medication use, or substance-use disorder

Adapted from American Academy of Sleep Medicine. International classification of sleep disorders. Diagnostic and coding manual. 2nd edition. Westchester (IL): American Academy of Sleep Medicine; 2005; with permission.

---

also be affected. Postpartum, OSA symptoms often improve or resolve.[19] In one series, the postpartum AHI reduced by one-third compared with the final trimester.[20] However, women with persistent OSA require follow-up because untreated OSA produces adverse health, mood, and social outcomes.

Mounting evidence illustrates the negative consequences of OSA on maternal-fetal health. Snoring and OSA in pregnancy are associated with increased risk of GDM,[6] preeclampsia,[18] and pregnancy-induced HTN (OR 7.5).[20] Even pregnant women with OSA symptoms who are not obese have a 6.6 OR for preeclampsia.[18] Cyclical hypoxemia and reoxygenation may promote proinflammatory markers that underlie these conditions. Habitual snoring is associated with increased cord blood levels of nucleated red blood cells, interleukin-6, and other inflammatory markers.[1,21] Future studies are needed to identify the frequency and severity of sleep-related breathing disturbance required to confer adverse pregnancy outcomes.

Prenatal care should include an assessment of sleep quality and a query on snoring and other symptoms of OSA. Habitual snoring in the setting of daytime problems, such as fatigue/sleepiness, witnessed apnea, or comorbidities (GDM, preeclampsia, HTN, obesity), should prompt evaluation. Standard screening tools are inadequate and pregnant patients with symptoms of OSA should be referred for a formal evaluation with PSG. Patients with OSA should be educated about the potential risks on maternal-fetal outcomes, course in pregnancy and postpartum, and treatment options. There is a scarcity of data to guide the treatment of OSA in pregnancy. Establishing the severity of OSA may provide a more clear treatment goal and plan. Early and aggressive treatment may be indicated even in mild OSA because the severity of disease required to adversely affect the fetus is unknown.

Conservative therapies should be recommended for all cases. These include behavioral modifications, such as using protective sleep positioning with the lateral sleeping position and/or head elevation, treatment of nasal congestion, and avoidance of sedatives, alcohol, excessive weight gain, and sleep deprivation. The first-line therapy for moderate to severe OSA is positive airway pressure (PAP) therapy, which can be delivered continuously (CPAP), by auto-titrating devices (AutoPAP), or bilevel delivery (Bilevel-PAP). Positive pressure therapy seems to be well tolerated during pregnancy.[22] The therapeutic pressure setting is usually established by a titration study performed in the sleep laboratory. Because of the enlarging gravid uterus and weight gain, pressure needs increase over time in pregnant women.[22] Other treatments, such as oral appliances, have not been studied in pregnancy but may be an effective alternative to PAP in appropriately chosen patients with mild OSA. The presence and severity of OSA should be reassessed postpartum because some women may no longer require treatment whereas others may benefit from a change in therapy that may improve long-term adherence. Studies evaluating CPAP during pregnancy show promising effects on blood presssure.[22] Further studies are needed to assess the effect of PAP therapy on other outcomes, effective evaluation methods, and therapeutic options in pregnancy and postpartum.

NARCOLEPSY AND HYPERSOMNIA

Hypersomnia, or excessive daytime sleepiness (EDS), is defined as the inability to maintain a wakeful and alert state during the usual waking portion of the day.[7] Severe hypersomnia is the hallmark of a group of central nervous system disorders including

Table 3
Classification and diagnostic criteria for narcolepsy with and without cataplexy

Classification	Diagnostic Criteria	
A. Narcolepsy without cataplexy	1.	Complaints of EDS occurring nearly daily for 3 mo or longer; and EDS is not otherwise explained by another sleep, medical, or mental disorder
	2.	Confirm with sleep testing: Nocturnal PSG followed by an MSLT
		a. PSG demonstrates sufficient nocturnal sleep (minimum of 6 h)
		b. MSLT demonstrates a mean sleep latency of ≤8 min and 2 or more Sleep Onset REM Periods
	3.	No cataplexy identified
B. Narcolepsy with cataplexy	1.	Meets criteria for number A1 above
	2.	In addition, there is the presence of cataplexy:
		a. Cataplexy is a sudden transient episode of weakness resulting from a loss of muscle tone that must be triggered by strong emotions, usually by positive emotion, such as laughing. It is generally bilateral, brief, and associated with a transient loss of deep tendon reflexes during the episode.
	3.	Where possible, confirm testing (as in A2 above)

Abbreviation: MSLT, Multiple Sleep Latency Test.
Adapted from American Academy of Sleep Medicine. International classification of sleep disorders. Diagnostic and coding manual. 2nd edition. Westchester (IL): American Academy of Sleep Medicine; 2005; with permission.

Table 4
Pharmacotherapy for narcolepsy

Drug Class and Names (Propriety)	Dosage (mg/d)	Food and Drug Administration Labeling	Pregnancy Class	Comments
Central Nervous Stimulants				
Methylphenidate: Short acting: (Ritalin, Metadate, Methylin); Intermediate acting: (Ritalin SR, Metadate ER, Methylin ER); Long acting: (Concerta, Metadate CD, Ritalin LA)	10–60	Narcolepsy[a]	C	Gastrointestinal distress, nervousness, palpitations, tics, headaches, insomnia
Dexmethylphenidate: Short acting: (Focalin) Long acting: (Focalin XR)	10–60			
Dextroamphetamines: Short acting: (Dexedrine, Dextrostat); Intermediate acting: (Dexedrine spansule); Dextrostat	5–60			Potential for abuse; risk of neonatal toxicity, arrhythmias and other stimulant effects
Mixed Dextro and Amphetamine Salts: Short acting: (Adderall); Long acting (Adderall XR)	5–60			
Methamphetamines: (Desoxyn)	5–40			
Non-Stimulants				
Modafinil (Provigil)	100–400	Narcolepsy, and other EDS	C	Headaches, nausea, and nervousness
Armodafinil (Nuvigil)	150–250			
Sodium oxybate (Xyrem): administered in 2 divided nightly doses	4.5–9 g	EDS and cataplexy of narcolepsy	B	Nausea, fluid retention, respiratory depression
Selective Serotonin Reuptake Inhibitors				
Fluoxetine (Prozac)	20–80	Cataplexy (off-label)	C	Insomnia, sexual dysfunction, dry mouth, nausea, headache
Venlafaxine (Effexor)	75–225			
Tricyclic Anti-Depressants				
Clomipramine (Anafranil)	10–200	Cataplexy (off-label)	C	Dry mouth, urinary retention, constipation, sexual dysfunction, orthostatic hypotension
Protriptyline (Vivactil)	5–30			
Desipramine (Norpramin, Pertofrane)	2–200			
Imipramine (Tofranil, Janimine)	25–200			

[a] Methylphenidate and amphetamines are indicated for the treatment of narcolepsy with specific mention of narcolepsy symptoms. Newer drug formulations comprising these compounds are not FDA approved specifically for narcolepsy.

narcolepsy. Narcolepsy affects an estimated 0.02% of the population.[7] Narcolepsy is characterized by a pentad of hypersomnia, disturbed nocturnal sleep, sleep-related hallucinations, sleep paralysis, and cataplexy, as a result of an inability of the wake and sleep promoting pathways in the brain to stabilize the sleep-wake cycle. The diagnostic criteria for narcolepsy are shown in **Table 3**.

Drug therapy for narcolepsy targets EDS and associated symptoms (**Table 4**). Management during pregnancy is limited by a paucity of data and treatment strategies that are largely based on case reports. According to practice parameters, modafinil and sodium oxybate are effective wake-promoting agents and are standards of therapy in the general population.[23] Armodafinil has recently been approved with similar efficacy. The traditional stimulants (eg, amphetamines, D-amphetamines, and methylphenidate) have a long history of clinical utility but the toxicity/teratogenicity is unknown. Alternatively, sodium oxybate is the only pregnancy class B agent and warrants consideration. Usage of wake-promoting agents during pregnancy and breastfeeding should be discussed carefully regarding the risks and benefits on a case-by-case basis. Some women may elect to take leave from work and discontinue driving for safety provisions while off medications.[24] In some patients, the safety risks of EDS (such as with driving) outweigh the risk of therapy. Some choose to simply reduce medication dosage.[25] Long-term neonatal effects are unknown, but the benefit and safety afforded to the mother may outweigh theoretical risks. Postpartum, if there are strong concerns regarding fetal transmission, a mother may elect to bottle-feed.

Significant cataplexy may affect labor and delivery. Reports of labor-induced cataplexy have lead to the need for cesarean delivery.[25] In narcoleptic patients with significant cataplexy, elective cesarean delivery should be considered after discussion with the sleep physician and obstetrician. Treatment with sodium oxybate is the only Federal Drug Administration-approved treatment for cataplexy. Agents, such as the tricyclic antidepressants and selective serotonin reuptake inhibitors may be used for the treatment of cataplexy but are off-label.

In contrast to the low prevalence of narcolepsy in the general and pregnant population, nonspecific hypersomnia commonly affects pregnant women. The Epworth Sleepiness Scale (ESS) is a widely used sleepiness scale that objectively measures sleepiness. Abnormal sleepiness (ESS $\geq$10) and napping is reported in most pregnant women.[2] Most daytime impairment from hypersomnia is reported in the first trimester.[2] Sleepiness may also be a consequence of other sleep disorders, such as OSA.

SUMMARY

Sleep and its associated disorders are profoundly affected by pregnancy and warrant evaluation in clinical practice. Although some changes in sleep may be physiologic, attention to the onset of sleep disorders in pregnant women is recommended. All pregnant women should be educated about the importance of sleep and avoidance of sleep deprivation. Evaluation and treatment of sleep disorders, especially OSA, may significantly affect maternal-fetal health outcomes.

REFERENCES

1. Facco FL, Kramer J, Ho KH, et al. Sleep disturbances in pregnancy. Obstet Gynecol 2010;115(1):77–83.
2. Neau JP, Texier B, Ingrand P. Sleep and vigilance disorders in pregnancy. Eur Neurol 2009;62(1):23–9.

3. Wilson DL, Barnes M, Ellett L, et al. Decreased sleep efficiency, increase wake after sleep onset and increased cortical arousals in late pregnancy. Aust N Z J Obstet Gynaecol 2011;51(1):38–46.

4. Hedman C, Pohjasvaara T, Tolonen U, et al. Effects of pregnancy on mothers' sleep. Sleep Med 2002;3(1):37–42.

5. Williams MA, Miller RS, Qiu C, et al. Associations of early pregnancy sleep duration with trimester-specific blood pressures and hypertensive disorders in pregnancy. Sleep 2010;33(10):1363–71.

6. Facco FL, Grobman WA, Kramer J, et al. Self-reported short sleep duration and frequent snoring in pregnancy: impact on glucose metabolism. Am J Obstet Gynecol 2010;203(2):142.e1–5.

7. American Academy of Sleep Medicine. International classification of sleep disorders. Diagnostic and coding manual. 2nd edition. Westchester (IL): American Academy of Sleep Medicine; 2005.

8. Swanson LM, Pickett SM, Flynn H, et al. Relationships among depression, anxiety and insomnia symptoms in perinatal women seeking mental health treatment. J Womens Health 2011;20(4):553–8.

9. Tamura H, Nakamura Y, Terron MP, et al. Melatonin and pregnancy in the human. Reprod Toxicol 2008;25(3):291–303.

10. Morin CM, Hauri PJ, Espie CA, et al. Nonpharmacologic treatment of chronic insomnia. An American Academy of Sleep Medicine review. Sleep 1999;22(8): 1134–56.

11. Beddoe AE, Lee KA, Weiss SJ, et al. Effects of mindful yoga on sleep in pregnant women: a pilot study. Biol Res Nurs 2010;11(4):363–70.

12. Manconi M, Govoni V, De Vito A, et al. Restless legs syndrome and pregnancy. Neurology 2004;63(6):1065–9.

13. Neau JP, Porcheron A, Mathis S, et al. Restless legs syndrome and pregnancy: a questionnaire study in the poitiers district, France. Eur Neurol 2010;64(5): 268–74.

14. Winkleman JW, Shahar E, Sharief I, et al. Association of restless legs syndrome and cardiovascular disease in the Sleep Heart Health Study. Neurology 2008; 70(1):35–42.

15. Dzaja A, Wehrle R, Lancel M, et al. Elevated estradiol plasma levels in women with restless legs during pregnancy. Sleep 2009;32(2):169–74.

16. Silber MH, Ehrenberg BL, Allen RP, et al. An algorithm for the management of restless legs syndrome. Mayo Clin Proc 2004;79(7):916–22.

17. Bartell S, Zallek S. Intravenous magnesium sulfate may relieve restless legs syndrome in pregnancy. J Clin Sleep Med 2006;2(2):187–8.

18. Olivarez SA, Ferres M, Antony K, et al. Obstructive sleep apnea screening in pregnancy, perinatal outcomes, and impact of maternal obesity. Am J Perinatol 2011;28(8):651–8.

19. Pien GW, Fife D, Pack AI, et al. Changes in symptoms of sleep-disordered breathing during pregnancy. Sleep 2005;28(10):1299–305.

20. Champagne K, Schwartzman K, Opatrny L, et al. Obstructive sleep apnoea and its association with gestational hypertension. Eur Respir J 2009;33(3):559–65.

21. Tauman R, Many A, Deutsch V, et al. Maternal snoring during pregnancy is associated with enhanced fetal erythropoiesis–a preliminary study. Sleep Med 2011; 12(5):518–22.

22. Guilleminault C, Palombini L, Poyares D, et al. Pre-eclampsia and nasal CPAP: part 1. Early intervention with nasal CPAP in pregnant women with risk factors for pre-eclampsia: preliminary findings. Sleep Med 2007;9(1):9–14.

23. Morgenthaler TI, Kapur VK, Brown T, et al. Practice parameters for the treatment of narcolepsy and other hypersomnias of central origin. Sleep 2007;30(12): 1705–11.

24. Hoque R, Chesson AL Jr. Conception, pregnancy, delivery, and breastfeeding in a narcoleptic patient with cataplexy. J Clin Sleep Med 2008;4(6):601–3.

25. Soltanifar S, Russell R. Neuraxial anaesthesia for caesarean section in a patient with narcolepsy and cataplexy. Int J Obstet Anesth 2010;19(4):440–3.

Pregnancy and Brain Tumors

Christopher M. Bonfield, MD, Johnathan A. Engh, MD*

KEYWORDS

- Pregnancy • Brain tumor • Management

KEY POINTS

- Brain tumors are uncommon in pregnant patients.
- Women of childbearing age with brain tumors require specific counseling about the medical risks of pregnancy as determined by the histology, location, and biologic characteristics of their tumor.
- Magnetic resonance imaging is safe in pregnancy, though scans are generally performed without intravenous contrast.
- Pregnancy is generally not a contraindication to surgical resection or brain tumor biopsy, although it is often a contraindication to radiation therapy and always a contraindication to systemic chemotherapy.
- Because of potential increase of intracranial pressure during Valsalva maneuver in a patient with a brain tumor, cesarean section is usually preferable to vaginal delivery once the fetus is term or near term.

INTRODUCTION

The first published report of a brain tumor diagnosed in a pregnant patient was written by Bernard[1] in 1898. It was recognized more than 100 years ago as a complex problem, and remains as such today.

The diagnosis of a brain tumor is a life-changing and stressful event for patients and their families. Treatment can be long and complex and often requires a multidisciplinary approach including a team of physicians from different specialties versed in varying modalities of therapy. These challenges are amplified if the patient is an expectant mother. Consideration of risks incurred from diagnostic tests and surveillance imaging, as well as treatments such as medication, surgery, radiation therapy (RT), and chemotherapy, must be considered for both mother and fetus. This article highlights the major issues and provides an overview to the care of the pregnant patient with a brain tumor, including diagnosis, clinical management, and follow-up issues.

Conflict of interest: The authors have nothing to disclose.
Department of Neurological Surgery, University of Pittsburgh Medical Center, 200 Lothrop Street, Suite B-400, Pittsburgh, PA 15213, USA
* Corresponding author.
E-mail address: enghja@upmc.edu

Neurol Clin 30 (2012) 937–946
doi:10.1016/j.ncl.2012.04.003
0733-8619/12/$ – see front matter © 2012 Elsevier Inc. All rights reserved.

neurologic.theclinics.com

INCIDENCE

According to the most recent cancer database statistics of the Center for Disease Control's National Program of Cancer Registries (NPCR),[2] brain cancer is a rare disease, especially compared with lung or breast cancer. For women of reproductive age (age 20–39 years, all races), the reported annual incidence is 2.0 to 3.2 new cases per 100,000 people. This incidence places brain cancer outside the 10 most common cancers in that population. However, mortality from the disease is 0.5 to 1.1 deaths per 100,000 people, placing brain tumors as the ninth most common cause of cancer-related death in this age group.

In 1988, Simon[3] proposed a probability-based calculation to determine the prevalence of brain tumors in pregnancy. He concluded that, in the United States, there were approximately 90 women each year who harbor a brain tumor while pregnant.[3] However, this was published before the widespread use of magnetic resonance imaging (MRI) and likely underestimates the true number of cases.

In most studies, it is reported that the relative frequency of the different primary brain tumor types is not changed by pregnancy. Furthermore, the incidence of brain tumors that become symptomatic during pregnancy seems to be decreased compared with that in age-matched women.[4] Whether this phenomenon is related to increased serum levels of circulating endogenous steroids during pregnancy or some alternative phenomenon is not known.

PRESENTATION

Intracranial neoplasms usually present with nonspecific symptoms such as headache, nausea, or vomiting, and focal neurologic deficits such as visual changes, hemiparesis, or seizures. This presentation is confounded in pregnancy, because many of the routine conditions in pregnancy are symptoms that could also be caused by increased intracranial pressure. It is therefore important for the clinician to be vigilant and have a low threshold to pursue imaging in a patient with prolonged, more severe, worsening, or nonremitting symptoms during pregnancy. It is recommended that any pregnant patient with a new neurologic deficit, without an otherwise known cause, receives a full evaluation by a qualified neurologist, and potentially undergoes intracranial imaging.

Many presenting symptoms of brain tumors are nonspecific and related to an increase in intracranial pressure secondary to mass effect of the tumor. In addition, the hypervolemic state produced in pregnancy by intravascular volume expansion and water retention can potentially exacerbate an already increased intracranial pressure. Headaches are the initial presenting symptom of brain tumor in approximately 36% to 90% of patients.[5] This is perhaps the hardest symptom to determine whether or not more work-up is necessary, because headaches are common in the general population as well as in pregnant women. However, certain characteristics of the headache are more concerning than others. New-onset headaches in women without a history of such headaches should be examined in greater detail. Headaches associated with increased intracranial pressure are usually gradual in onset, with a course that is continually worsening over time. They are routinely daily headaches and are often worse in the morning, or with maneuvers that increase intracranial pressure, such as lying down, coughing, exertion, or bearing down. If a headache fits these criteria, it is recommended that further work-up be completed.

Nausea and vomiting are nonspecific symptoms of brain tumors and increased intracranial pressure. Common in pregnancy, like headaches, these symptoms can be attributed to routine morning sickness or the more severe condition of hyperemesis gravidarum. Approximately 25% of patients with brain tumors are observed to have nausea and vomiting.[6] In most pregnant women, the nausea and vomiting are worst in the first trimester. New-onset nausea and vomiting in the second and third trimester, after the morning sickness has usually resolved, especially in patients without such symptoms in their pregnancy thus far, should be closely investigated.

Pregnancy is both a mental and physiologic burden on the patient. The body is supporting growth of the fetus, and the mother's body can be physically stressed, leading to severe fatigue. However, in a patient with considerable drowsiness or a frank change in level of consciousness, medical attention should be sought, and intracranial imaging should be performed in such cases.

Some tumors, especially in the occipital cortex or in the sellar region, can present with visual symptoms. There have been many documented cases of pregnant patients with pituitary tumors who develop new visual field defects.[7,8] This is may be caused by a rapid increase in the size of the tumor, but is more often caused by normal physiologic expansion of the pituitary gland, which causes compression of the optic apparatus in the setting of an associated tumor. In addition, many of these deficits resolve after delivery, so acute treatment may not be necessary in all cases.

Approximately 30% to 50% of brain tumors present with a new-onset seizure and 10% to 30% develop seizures during the disease course.[9] A seizure secondary to a mass is likely to have a focal onset, with the possibility of generalization. A new seizure should always warrant a work-up. However, seizures that are generalized in onset and occur in the second or early third trimester may also be related to eclampsia and should be evaluated and treated as such.[10]

DIAGNOSIS

The diagnosis of a brain tumor requires imaging, either computed tomography (CT; or computed axial tomography [CAT]) or MRI. In the setting of pregnancy, MRI is the preferred imaging modality because of its greater resolution, increased sensitivity, and lack of ionizing radiation. MRI scanning without intravenous contrast has been shown to be safe for both the mother and the fetus.[11] CT imaging can also be useful for the initial diagnosis of a brain tumor. Its lower cost, faster scan time, and greater availability are all distinct advantages compared with MRI. However, it has lower resolution and uses ionizing radiation to acquire the images. Despite this, many studies have shown that cranial CT scanning is safe for the fetus, especially in the setting of abdominal lead shielding techniques.[3] CT scanning may be the only available imaging modality at some centers. If the clinical suspicion of a brain mass is high, imaging should not be foregone because of the presence of a CT scanner and no MRI available.

Administration of intravenous (IV) contrast enhances the diagnostic yield of cranial imaging. Iodinated contrast used in CT scanning has the potential to cause nephrotoxicity and allergy-related side effects to all patients. However, it has not been shown to directly cause birth defects. There are reports that the IV dye can rarely cause hypothyroidism in the fetus.[12] Therefore, neonatal thyroid function should be checked during the first week of life in these patients. MRI contrast is gadolinium based, and has a better side effect profile than CT contrast. It has a lower propensity to cause an allergic reaction and does not cause nephrotoxicity. The MRI contrast can cross the placenta, but has not been shown to cause birth defects in the fetus.[13,14] Despite these reports, imaging can still be controversial and a discussion should be had with the radiology department who will be acquiring the images to discuss the patient, what type of imaging will be pursued, and whether contrast will be given for that specific study. The appropriate information can usually be gleaned from noncontrasted MRI scans to guide therapy in pregnant patients, which keeps fetal risk at a minimum.

A good ophthalmologic examination can also be beneficial in the diagnosis of intracranial tumors. Visual deficits can be found on detailed visual acuity testing or at the bedside. This evaluation is especially important to those who have known pituitary tumors diagnosed before pregnancy. In addition, papilledema is a manifestation of increased intracranial pressure and can be used as a noninvasive diagnostic tool when deciding whether nonspecific symptoms such as headache or nausea and vomiting should warrant imaging.

Serum tests can also add vital information during the diagnostic phase, especially in pituitary tumors, in which serum tests may diagnose a secreting tumor or help to monitor endocrine function. However, hormonal levels fluctuate during pregnancy and do not have the same expected levels compared with nonpregnant states. In addition, in the setting of pineal region tumors, imaging and serum markers may facilitate the diagnosis of a nongerminomatous germ cell tumor without a requirement for biopsy.

MANAGEMENT

The management of brain tumors is complex and often requires a combination of medical and surgical techniques. No single technique is perfect and, as always, the risks of the therapy (both to the mother and the fetus) have to be weighed against the potential benefit. In these cases, the principle guiding treatment is usually to treat the mother with the therapy that would be recommended in the absence of pregnancy, then to tailor the approach as necessary to minimize fetal risk. The best therapy for the mother is usually the best therapy for the fetus.

Medical management of brain tumors can be used either to treat the tumor, or to treat the condition and symptoms until delivery, after which definitive treatment can be given. The most important component of medical therapy in this setting is steroids. Steroids alleviate vasogenic edema surrounding a tumor, which can facilitate neurologic recovery. In addition, steroids facilitate surfactant formation in the fetal lung, making an early delivery both safer and more feasible. Despite these benefits, long-term steroid use can lead to adrenal insufficiency in the developing fetus.[15] However, this is uncommon, and steroid use has the potential to delay surgery, chemotherapy, or RT until after the baby is safely delivered. Therefore, we generally advocate judicious use of steroid therapy to treat symptomatic brain tumors in the setting of pregnancy.

Antiepileptic drugs (AEDs) are also commonly used to treat patients with brain tumors, but are more controversial than steroids in the setting of pregnancy. Many AEDs are documented teratogens, and the others are of indeterminate risk.[16] However, it is widely accepted that the risk of harm from repeated seizures outweighs the potential side effects from the medication, including potential teratogenicity. In general, the authors advocate using AEDs in the setting of documented seizures in a pregnant patient, but not for seizure prophylaxis in the absence of symptoms. Medical guidance from an epileptologist is helpful in such cases.

Conventional chemotherapy should be delayed until after delivery in most instances, because of the fetal risk. However, some medications to treat pituitary tumors seem to be safe for the pregnant patient and have the potential to delay or obviate surgical resection of the tumor. In prolactin-secreting pituitary tumors, bromocriptine and dopamine analogues have acceptable safety profiles,[17] but should be used sparingly in breastfeeding mothers. In addition, octreotide seems to be acceptably safe for pregnant patients with acromegaly. In addition, local chemotherapy using carmustine-impregnated wafers has been reported as a safe option for pregnant patients requiring glioma resection.[18] However, standard systemic glioma treatments, such as temozolomide and bevacizumab, are generally not administered during pregnancy.

RT has the potential to cause mental retardation, congenital defects, and childhood malignancies, especially if given in the first trimester. However, if necessary, the risk to the fetus can be decreased if the RT is given in the second or third trimesters. Limiting the dose,[19] maximizing the plan to avoid fetus exposure, using abdominal lead shielding, and changing the position of the patient during the therapy[20] are reported ways to limit radiation to the fetus and to prevent unwanted side effects as well. This therapy is generally limited to rare cases. Stereotactic radiosurgery, using instruments such as the Gamma Knife (Elekta Inc., Stockholm, Sweden) or Cyber Knife (Accuray Inc., Sunnyvale, CA, USA) is a safer method to provide focal radiation treatment, because the fetal radiation exposure is nearly zero using such techniques.

Surgical resection is also frequently used in the treatment of brain tumors, especially in the setting of a large tumor, significant mass effect causing symptoms, or a high-grade, aggressive lesion. Craniotomy can be undertaken if the mass effect on critical structures necessitates immediate treatment. In certain circumstances, this may be completed under local anesthesia and IV sedation. General anesthesia is also acceptable. In addition, stereotactic biopsy under local anesthesia to obtain a tissue diagnosis is a reasonable option before the start of RT. Intraoperative considerations must also be made. It is important that the maternal-fetal medicine service is aware, and most recommend fetal monitoring during the operation. Positioning of the patient may also have to be adjusted. For example, a sitting or lateral position should be used instead of placing the patient prone.[21]

Alterations must be made in the postoperative period as well. Intermittent, but increased, fetal monitoring may be necessary. Pain control should be achieved, but with knowledge of which drugs have greater potential to cause the fetus harm. Imaging may be necessary, but ionizing radiation and contrast agents should be avoided.

Treatment may also depend on the timing of presentation. If the patient is in her first trimester, a therapeutic abortion may be offered. In such cases, the risk of treatment, whether surgery, RT, or chemotherapy, may be too great to the fetus, and a delay in treatment may be unsafe for the mother. For those patients within the third trimester, and with tumors without emergent treatment needs, it may be possible to delay treatment until after delivery, or to facilitate cesarean delivery before therapy.

When an expecting mother with a stable tumor is pending delivery, a question that is often asked is how best to deliver the fetus (vaginal vs cesarean delivery). In general, the authors favor cesarean delivery in such cases, to avoid the inevitable increases in intracranial pressure incurred by vaginal delivery. In addition, general anesthesia is a preferred option rather than spinal or epidural anesthesia, because a cerebrospinal fluid (CSF) leak can lead to severe neurologic morbidity in the setting of an intracranial mass lesion. In the authors' experience, scheduled cesarean delivery under general anesthesia following documentation of fetal lung maturity is the safest procedure in such cases.

For low-grade, slow-growing, or benign tumors, it may be feasible to observe the tumor throughout pregnancy. In these cases, it is important to follow the patient's neurologic examination, and may also be beneficial to obtain routine laboratory work or surveillance imaging depending on the tumor type. Noncontrasted MRI imaging is generally preferred.

It is also important to counsel the patients with known brain tumors about the risks of becoming pregnant. In these instances, it may be beneficial to have the tumor treated before pregnancy to avoid the potential risks of the treatments or the tumor becoming more aggressive during pregnancy. Such decisions are best handled on a case-by-case basis. For example, a 32-year-old woman with a recently resected meningioma without atypical features is a safer candidate for pregnancy than the same patient in remission following temozolomide and RT for an anaplastic astrocytoma.

TUMOR TYPES

No specific type of brain tumor seems to have a different incidence in the setting of pregnancy. However, because of the hormonal and physiologic changes incurred during pregnancy, some tumors can be affected during that time. As in nonpregnant women of the same age, gliomas and meningiomas are the 2 most common types.[4] However, numerous other tumors have now been reported in the literature, and each carries with it its own specific considerations for diagnosis and treatment. This article reviews some of the more common tumor types seen in pregnancy and discusses their individual characteristics.

The most common primary intraparenchymal brain tumors in adults are gliomas. These tumors are intrinsic parenchymal tumors that arise from glial cells, which, depending on the grade, can be slow growing or aggressive and invasive. These tumors typically present with nonspecific symptoms like headache or nausea and vomiting. They can also cause seizures or focal neurologic deficits. For reasons that are not clear, gliomas seem to present more often during the first 2 trimesters.[22] Low-grade gliomas (astrocytoma or oligodendroglioma) are routinely slow growing and indolent. Surgical resection can usually be delayed until after delivery. RT is often added as an adjunct therapy for astrocytomas and chemotherapy for oligodendrogliomas in the postpartum phase. Steroids are routinely used as a temporizing measure by decreasing the peritumoral edema, and AEDs can prevent seizures. However, because of the hypervolemic state of pregnancy, the cerebral edema can worsen during pregnancy and cause the patient's symptoms to worsen. Immediate surgical resection is usually only needed for large tumors with significant mass effect or those with refractory seizures.

High-grade gliomas (anaplastic astrocytoma and glioblastoma multiforme) are more common and more malignant. They typically produce more inflammation and edema and cause a more significant and faster neurologic deterioration. The prognosis is poor and the patient's condition can worsen quickly. In this case, surgery should not be postponed for a prolonged length of time. If the fetus is viable or the delivery is imminent, it is reasonable to induce labor or schedule a caesarian section. Otherwise, with careful planning, a craniotomy can be performed safely. Local chemotherapy placed in the tumor bed during surgery, such as carmustine-impregnated wafers, seems safe,[18] but further chemotherapy or RT should be delayed until after delivery.

Meningiomas are the most common benign brain tumor.[23] They originate from arachnoid cap cells in the meninges surrounding the brain and are slow growing and cause symptoms by local mass effect. Meningiomas tend to present more often during the third trimester and pregnancy does not seem to cause an increase in incidence.[22] However, pregnancy may affect size and growth because of hormonal effects (70%–90% have progesterone and 33%–38% estrogen receptors)[10] and a hypervolemic state. In most instances, resection is able to be deferred until after delivery, and steroids and AEDs are used if needed. There is no need for RT or stereotactic radiosurgery during pregnancy. Symptoms from small, previously undiagnosed meningiomas usually resolve after pregnancy; however, they can recur with subsequent pregnancies. Therefore, the tumor should probably be treated before any additional planned pregnancies.

Acoustic neuromas are another common benign tumor that arises from the vestibular portion of the vestibulocochlear nerve (eighth cranial nerve). Common symptoms are tinnitus, hearing loss, and imbalance. Similar to meningiomas, the growth of acoustic neuromas may be affected by hormonal alterations seen in pregnancy.[24] There does not seem to be an increase in incidence. Resection should be delayed until postpartum if possible. There is generally no role for stereotactic radiosurgery during pregnancy for such tumors.

Pituitary tumors are often seen, and frequently diagnosed, in pregnant patients. It is reported that approximately 5% to 15% of people with known pituitary tumors can have tumor growth during pregnancy, some of which require treatment, especially those with early symptoms, rapid progression, or apoplexy.[25] The pituitary gland enlarges during pregnancy because of estrogen-stimulated hyperplasia and hypertrophy of prolactin-producing lactotropes. If the gland is already large because of a mass, the physiologic enlargement can cause enough growth to cause symptoms. These patients can present with headache, visual deficits, or endocrine dysfunction. Breastfeeding may also induce tumor growth.[10] Most tumors regress after pregnancy and lactation are completed; as a result, symptoms abate. Treatment is specific depending on the type of pituitary tumor. However, the authors offer the following general guidelines: if the tumor is a microadenoma (<1 cm) and asymptomatic, observation is usually adequate. If the tumor is a macroadenoma (>1 cm) and symptomatic, a trial of bromocriptine (which reduces the hypertrophied lactotropes) is a reasonable first-line therapy, followed by surgery if the medical treatment fails. Serum hormone levels should also be checked, both before and during treatment, to aid in the diagnosis of the specific type of tumor and to follow treatment response.

Pregnancy alone can increase the serum prolactin level by a factor of 10[8]; therefore, an increased prolactin level is not necessarily caused by a prolactinoma. In addition, treatment of a prolactinoma is often a prerequisite for pregnancy. These tumors are usually treated with bromocriptine (or another dopamine analogue) and surgical resection, if needed. However, for those tumors not entirely treated before pregnancy, or for women who become pregnant during treatment, further therapy may be warranted. If the tumor is a microadenoma (<1 cm), the patient can usually be followed clinically for symptoms, undergo serial visual examinations, and have scheduled surveillance MRI scans. Bromocriptine, although it has a favorable safety profile, can be stopped if the tumor is small and stable, but can be restarted if tumor growth is noted. Macroadenomas (>1 cm) should be treated before pregnancy, if possible. However, if they present during pregnancy, first-line treatment is usually bromocriptine, followed by surgery if necessary.[17]

Less common pituitary tumors have also been described in the setting of pregnancy. The treatment of Cushing disease (an adrenocorticotropic hormone–producing tumor) is usually surgical resection of the tumor. In the setting of acromegaly (a growth hormone–producing tumor), medical treatment is warranted first with bromocriptine with or without octreotide, only followed with surgery if the medical management is unsuccessful.[26]

Colloid cysts have also been reported in pregnant women. These masses originate in the roof of the anterior third ventricle and can cause symptoms of hydrocephalus by blocking CSF outflow from the lateral ventricles at the foramina of Monroe. In nonpregnant patients, the most common presenting symptom is headache, but vertigo,

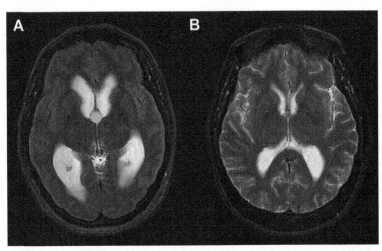

Fig. 1. Case Study: A 38-year-old woman presents with headache, confusion, gait instability, and vomiting while 33 weeks pregnant. (*A*) T2-weighted axial MRI shows a 12-mm colloid cyst of the third ventricle with hydrocephalus and transependymal flow of CSF. Because of the pregnancy and the fluid signal characteristics of the cyst, a CT-guided stereotactic cyst aspiration was performed using intravenous sedation. A normal fetus was delivered vaginally at term. (*B*) One-year after surgery, the same MRI protocol shows a 7-mm cyst with resolution of hydrocephalus. The patient remains asymptomatic.

syncope, lethargy, and, in rare cases, sudden death can occur if foraminal obstruction is severe. These tumors can routinely be observed if less than 7 mm in size or asymptomatic; however, larger masses and those with hydrocephalus may need urgent surgical resection or CSF diversion such as shunting.[27] In our institution, we have also performed stereotactic aspiration of a colloid cyst under local anesthesia and IV sedation to avoid a longer, riskier surgery under general anesthesia (**Fig. 1**).

Metastatic tumors, from primary sites like breast or lung, are the most common brain tumors in adults, but are rare in pregnant women. However, metastatic choriocarcinoma has been described.[28] This condition is a general trophoblastic disease that may develop after molar pregnancy, abortion, ectopic pregnancy, or term pregnancy. These tumors have a tendency to hemorrhage. Patients diagnosed with systemic choriocarcinoma should have screening MRI at diagnosis, because approximately 20% have metastatic disease to the brain. Serum levels of β-human chorionic gonadotropin can also be checked. Treatment with RT and chemotherapy can begin immediately, because there is no viable fetus present.

Other tumor types have also been described in the literature in the setting of pregnancy, including craniopharyngioma,[29] ependymoma,[30] hemangioblastoma,[31] pineal region tumor,[22] medulloblastoma,[32] primary central nervous system lymphoma,[33] paraglanglioma,[34] primary meningeal sarcoma,[35] and dysembryoplastic neuroepithelial tumor.[36] Therapy varies depending on the tumor, but follows the general principles of treatment discussed earlier.

SUMMARY

Brain tumors in the setting of pregnancy are challenging because of a combination of factors including difficulties in diagnosis, nuances of maternal physiology, fetal toxicity and viability, and complexity of interventions. In general, treatment is performed for symptomatic lesions, with care to minimize toxicity to both mother and fetus. Multidisciplinary input from maternal-fetal medicine, anesthesiology, neurosurgery, and sometimes neurology is necessary to achieve good outcomes. Treatment is best allocated on a case-by-case basis.

REFERENCES

1. Bernard MH. Rapid evolution of cerebral sarcoma during the course of pregnancy and the after effects of childbirth. Obstet Soc Paris Bull 1898;1:296–8.
2. Centers for Disease Control National Program of Cancer Registries. Available at: http://www.cdc.gov/cancer/npcr. Accessed February 3, 2012.
3. Simon RH. Brain tumors in pregnancy. Semin Neurol 1988;8(3):214–21.
4. Roelvink NC, Kamphorst W, van Alphen HA, et al. Pregnancy-related primary brain and spinal tumors. Arch Neurol 1987;44(2):209–15.
5. Frishberg BM. Neuroimaging in presumed primary headache disorders. Semin Neurol 1997;17:373–82.
6. Chang CH, Horton J, Schoenfeld V, et al. Comparison of postoperative radiotherapy and combined postoperative radiotherapy and chemotherapy in the multidisciplinary management of malignant gliomas. A joint Radiation Therapy Oncology Group and Eastern Cooperative Oncology Group study. Cancer 1983;52:997–1007.
7. Jan M, Destrieux C. Pituitary disorders in pregnancy. Neurochirurgie 2000;46(2): 88–94.
8. Molitch ME. Pituitary tumors and pregnancy. Growth Horm IGF Res 2003; 13(Suppl A):S38–44.
9. van Breemen MS, Wilms EB, Vecht CJ. Epilepsy in patients with brain tumours: epidemiology, mechanisms, and management. Lancet Neurol 2007;6(5):421–30.
10. DeAngelis LM. Central nervous system neoplasms in pregnancy. Adv Neurol 1994;64:139–52.
11. Levine D, Barnes PD, Madsen JR, et al. Central nervous system abnormalities assessed with prenatal magnetic resonance imaging. Obstet Gynecol 1999;94: 1011–9.
12. Webb JA, Thomsen HS, Morcos SK. The use of iodinated and gadolinium contrast media during pregnancy and lactation. Eur Radiol 2005;15(6):1234–40.
13. Edelman RR, Warach S. Magnetic resonance imaging. N Engl J Med 1993;328: 708–16.
14. Sundgren PC, Leander P. Is administration of gadolinium-based contrast media to pregnant women and small children justified? J Magn Reson Imaging 2011; 34(4):750–7.
15. Trainer PJ. Corticosteroids and pregnancy. Semin Reprod Med 2002;20(4): 375–80.
16. Klein AM. Epilepsy cases in pregnant and postpartum women: a practical approach. Semin Neurol 2011;31(4):392–6.
17. Imran SA, Ur E, Clarke DB. Managing prolactin-secreting adenomas during pregnancy. Can Fam Physician 2007;53(4):653–8.
18. Stevenson CB, Thompson RC. The clinical management of intracranial neoplasms in pregnancy. Clin Obstet Gynecol 2005;48(1):24–37.
19. Mazonakis M, Damilakis J, Theoharopoulos N, et al. Brain radiotherapy during pregnancy: an analysis of conceptus dose using anthropomorphic phantoms. Br J Radiol 1999;72(855):274–8.

20. Magné N, Marcié S, Pignol JP, et al. Radiotherapy for a solitary brain metastasis during pregnancy: a method for reducing fetal dose. Br J Radiol 2001;74(883): 638–41.
21. Giannini A, Bricchi M. Posterior fossa surgery in the sitting position in a pregnant patient with cerebellopontine angle meningioma. Br J Anaesth 1999;82(6):941–4.
22. Cohen-Gadol AA, Friedman JA, Friedman JD, et al. Neurosurgical management of intracranial lesions in the pregnant patient: a 36-year institutional experience and review of the literature. J Neurosurg 2009;111(6):1150–7.
23. Marta GN, Correa SF, Teixeira MJ. Meningioma: review of the literature with emphasis on the approach to radiotherapy. Expert Rev Anticancer Ther 2011; 11(11):1749–58.
24. Allen J, Eldridge R, Koerber T, et al. Acoustic neuroma in the last months of pregnancy. Am J Obstet Gynecol 1974;119:516–20.
25. Iuliano S, Laws ER Jr. Management of pituitary tumors in pregnancy. Semin Neurol 2011;31(4):423–8.
26. Ben-Shlomo A, Melmed S. Acromegaly. Endocrinol Metab Clin North Am 2001;30: 565–83.
27. Pollock BE, Huston J 3rd. Natural history of asymptomatic colloid cysts of the third ventricle. J Neurosurg 1999;91(3):364–9.
28. Weed JC Jr, Hunter VJ. Diagnosis and management of brain metastasis from gestational trophoblastic disease. Oncology (Huntingt) 1991;5:48–50 [discussion: 50, 53–4].
29. Hiett AK, Barton JR. Diabetes insipidus associated with craniopharyngioma in pregnancy. Obstet Gynecol 1990;76(5 Pt 2):982–4.
30. Kamiński K, Bazowski P, Grzonka D, et al. Rare case of a malignant brain neoplasm in an 18-years old pregnant woman. Ginekol Pol 2003;74(6):472–4.
31. Naidoo K, Bhigjee AI. Multiple cerebellar haemangioblastomas symptomatic during pregnancy. Br J Neurosurg 1998;12(3):281–4.
32. Pollack RN, Pollak M, Rochon L. Pregnancy complicated by medulloblastoma with metastases to the placenta. Obstet Gynecol 1993;81(5 Pt 2):858–9.
33. Imai A, Kawabata I, Tamaya T. Primary brain malignant lymphoma newly diagnosed during pregnancy. J Med 1995;26(5-6):333–6.
34. Verstraeten PR, de Boer R. Pregnancy and functional paraganglioma. Eur J Obstet Gynecol Reprod Biol 1987;26(2):157–64.
35. Hong B, Hermann EJ, Hollwitz B, et al. Primary meningeal sarcoma with leiomyoblastic differentiation complicating pregnancy. Clin Neurol Neurosurg 2010; 112(6):516–9.
36. Terauchi M, Kubota T, Aso T, et al. Dysembryoplastic neuroepithelial tumor in pregnancy. Obstet Gynecol 2006;108(3 Pt 2):730–2.

Index

A

Abscess(es)
   epidural
      during labor and delivery
         anesthesia-related, 825–826
ACE inhibitors. *See* Angiotensin-converting enzyme (ACE) inhibitors
Acetaminophen
   for headaches during pregnancy and lactation, 849, 851
Acute inflammatory demyelinating polyradiculoneuropathy (AIDP)
   in pregnancy, 895–896
AFE. *See* Amniotic fluid embolism (AFE)
AIDP. *See* Acute inflammatory demyelinating polyradiculoneuropathy (AIDP)
ALS. *See* Amyotrophic lateral sclerosis (ALS)
Amniotic fluid embolism (AFE)
   during pregnancy
      imaging of, 804–805
      stroke due to, 918–919
Amyotrophic lateral sclerosis (ALS)
   in pregnancy, 904–905
Analgesics
   for headaches during pregnancy and lactation, 849–851
Anesthesia/anesthetics
   obstetric
      neurologic complications in patient receiving, **823–833**. *See also* Obstetric
         anesthesia, neurologic complications in patient receiving
Angiopathy
   postpartum
      during pregnancy
         imaging of, 803–804
Angiotensin-converting enzyme (ACE) inhibitors
   in headache prevention during pregnancy and lactation, 855, 860
Angiotensin II receptor antagonists
   in headache prevention during pregnancy and lactation, 855, 859
Anterior spinal artery syndrome
   during labor and delivery
      anesthesia-related, 826–827
Anti-inflammatory drugs
   nonsteroidal
      for headaches during pregnancy and lactation, 850, 851
Anticoagulants
   in stroke prevention during pregnancy, 920–921

Neurol Clin 30 (2012) 947–962
http://dx.doi.org/10.1016/S0733-8619(12)00035-7
0733-8619/12/$ – see front matter © 2012 Elsevier Inc. All rights reserved.

neurologic.theclinics.com

Antidepressants
   tricyclic
      in headache prevention during pregnancy and lactation, 854, 859
Antiemetics
   for headaches during pregnancy and lactation, 852–853, 857
Antiepileptics
   in headache prevention during pregnancy and lactation, 855–856, 860
   in women with epilepsy during postpartum period, 870–871
Antiplatelet therapy
   in stroke prevention during pregnancy, 920–921
Aspirin
   in headache management during pregnancy and lactation, 850, 851
   in headache prevention during pregnancy and lactation, 854, 858
Assisted reproduction techniques
   in MS patients, 879

B

Back pain
   during labor and delivery
      anesthesia-related, 829
   during pregnancy
      imaging of, 813–816
Barbiturates
   for headaches during pregnancy and lactation, 852, 857
Bell's palsy
   in pregnancy, 894
Birth trauma
   anesthesia-related, 830–831
   neuropathy due to
      diagnosis and management of, 831–832
β-Blockers
   in headache prevention during pregnancy and lactation, 855, 858–859
Body water
   during pregnancy
      stroke related to, 915
Botulinum toxin
   in headache prevention during pregnancy and lactation, 856, 860
Brain tumors
   during pregnancy, **937–946**
      described, 937
      diagnosis of, 939–940
      incidence of, 938
      management of, 940–942
      presentation of, 938–939
      types of, 942–944
Breastfeeding
   by MS patients, 883–884
   by women with epilepsy, 868–870
      pharmacokinetics of, 868–870
      psychosocial concerns related to, 868

Breathing
    sleep-disordered
        during pregnancy, 930–932

C

Calcium channel blockers
    in headache prevention during pregnancy and lactation, 855, 859
Carbamazepine
    in women with epilepsy during postpartum period, 871
Cardiomyopathy
    peripartum
        stroke due to, 918
Cardiovascular system
    pregnancy effects on, 781–783
        stroke related to, 915
Cauda equina syndrome
    during labor and delivery
        anesthesia-related, 827
CBF. See Cerebral blood flow (CBF)
Cerebral blood flow (CBF)
    preeclampsia in
        vs. physiologic changes in pregnancy, 782–783
Cerebral venous and sinus thrombosis (CVST)
    stroke due to, 917–918
Charcot-Marie-Tooth disease
    in pregnancy, 899–900
Choriocarcinoma
    stroke due to, 918
Chronic inflammatory demyelinating polyradiculoneuropathy (CIDP)
    in pregnancy, 896
CIDP. See Chronic inflammatory demyelinating polyradiculoneuropathy (CIDP)
Cluster headache
    during pregnancy
        effects of, 836–837
        investigations for, 849
Cognitive issues
    in women with epilepsy during postpartum period, 872
Common peroneal nerve injury
    birth trauma–related, 831
Computed tomography (CT)
    of brain during pregnancy, 919
Congenital nemaline rod myopathy
    in pregnancy, 902
Contraception
    in women with epilepsy during postpartum period, 874
Counseling
    pregnancy-related
        in MS patients, 882
CVST. See Cerebral venous and sinus thrombosis (CVST)

D

Depression
  in women with epilepsy during postpartum period, 873–874
Dihydroergotamine
  for headaches during pregnancy and lactation, 853, 858
Direct spinal cord injury
  during labor and delivery
    anesthesia-related, 824
Disease-modifying therapies (DMTs)
  for MS
    in pregnancy, 882
DMTs. *See* Disease-modifying therapies (DMTs)
Drug(s). *See also specific drugs and indications*
  in women with epilepsy during postpartum period, 870–872. *See also specific drugs and*
    Epilepsy, postpartum period in women with, drug dose adjustment

E

Eclampsia
  stroke due to, 915–916
Embolism
  amniotic fluid
    during pregnancy
      imaging of, 804–805
      stroke due to, 918–919
  paradoxic
    stroke due to, 919
Encephalopathy(ies)
  Wernicke
    during pregnancy
      imaging of, 805–806
Endocrine changes
  during pregnancy
    stroke related to, 915
Epidural abscess
  during labor and delivery
    anesthesia-related, 825–826
Epidural hematoma
  during labor and delivery
    anesthesia-related, 825
Epilepsy
  postpartum period in women with, **867–875**
    breastfeeding, 868–870
    case study, 867
    cognitive issues, 872
    contraception, 874
    depression, 873–874
    drug dose adjustment, 870–872
      antiepileptics, 870–871
      carbamazepine, 871

lamotrigine, 871
levetiracetam, 872
phenytoin, 871
topiramate, 872
valproic acid, 871
zonisamide, 872
safety issues, 872–873
during pregnancy
imaging of, 808
Ergot(s)
for headaches during pregnancy and lactation, 853, 858
Ergotamine
for headaches during pregnancy and lactation, 853, 858

F

Facioscapulohumeral muscular dystrophy (FSHD)
in pregnancy, 900
Femoral nerve injury
birth trauma–related, 831
Femoral neuropathy
in pregnancy, 893–894
Focal peripheral nerve and root lesions
postpartum foot drop due to
in pregnancy, 892–893
Foot drop
postpartum
focal peripheral nerve and root lesions–related
in pregnancy, 892–893
FSHD. *See* Facioscapulohumeral muscular dystrophy (FSHD)

G

Gabapentin
in headache prevention during pregnancy and lactation, 855, 860
Gastroesophageal sphincter
preeclampsia in
vs. physiologic changes in pregnancy, 784
Gastroesophageal system
pregnancy effects on, 785
Gestational trophoblastic disease
imaging of, 809
Guillain-Barré syndrome
in pregnancy, 895–896

H

HBPN. *See* Hereditary brachial plexus neuropathy (HBPN)
Headache(s). *See also specific types*
postdural puncture
during labor and delivery
anesthesia-related, 827–828

Headache(s) (*continued*)
  in pregnancy, **835–866**
    case study, 862
    cluster headache, 836–837
    described, 835–836
    investigations for, 846
    management of, 846–849
      emergency, 860–861
      nonpharmacologic, 847–848
      pharmacologic, 848–849
        analgesics, 849–851
        antiemetics, 852–853, 857
        barbiturates, 852, 857
        ergots, 853, 858
        opiates, 852, 857
        safety of, 849
        triptans, 853, 857–858
      prophylactic, 854–856, 858–860
        ACE inhibitors, 855, 860
        angiotensin II receptor antagonists, 855, 859
        antiepileptics, 855–856, 860
        aspirin, 854, 858
        β-blockers, 855, 858–859
        botulinum toxin, 856, 860
        calcium channel blockers, 855, 859
        lithium, 856, 860
        methylsergide, 856, 860
        SSRIs, 855, 859
        TCAs, 854, 859
    migraine, 836–841
    outcome of pregnancy effects, 842–843
    postpartum headache, 842
    tension-type headache, 836
      investigations for, 848–849
    vascular disorders associated with, 843–846
  prevalence of
    by type, 835
  primary
    effect on pregnancy and lactation, 842–846
    pregnancy and lactation effects of, 836–842
  secondary
    in pregnancy, 846
Hematologic system
  pregnancy effects on, 783
    stroke related to, 915
Hematoma(s)
  epidural
    during labor and delivery
      anesthesia-related, 825
Hemorrhage
  in pregnancy

treatment of, 922
subarachnoid
during pregnancy
imaging of, 796
Hereditary brachial plexus neuropathy (HBPN)
in pregnancy, 900
Hereditary neuropathy with liability to pressure palsies (HNPP)
in pregnancy, 900
HNPP. See Hereditary neuropathy with liability to pressure palsies (HNPP)
Hypersomnia
during pregnancy, 932–934
Hypophysitis
lymphocytic
during pregnancy
imaging of, 812–813
Hypotension
intracranial
during pregnancy
imaging of, 816

I

Idiopathic facial nerve palsy
in pregnancy, 894
Immunologic system
pregnancy effects on, 784–785
Inflammatory muscle disease
in pregnancy, 896–897
Insomnia
during pregnancy, 926–927
Intercostal neuralgia
in pregnancy, 895
Intracranial hypotension
during pregnancy
imaging of, 816

K

Kidney(s)
pregnancy effects on, 784

L

Labor and delivery
anesthesia during
neurologic complications in patient receiving, **823–833**. See also specific
complications and Obstetric anesthesia, neurologic complications in patient
receiving
in MS patients, 881
Lactation
drugs during
safety of, 849

Lactation (*continued*)
    headaches during, 842–846
        investigations for, 846
        management of, 846–849
Lamotrigine
    in women with epilepsy during postpartum period, 871
Lateral femoral cutaneous nerve injury
    birth trauma–related, 831
Lateral femoral cutaneous neuropathy
    in pregnancy, 891–892
Levetiracetam
    in women with epilepsy during postpartum period, 872
LGMDs. *See* Limb-girdle muscular dystrophies (LGMDs)
Limb-girdle muscular dystrophies (LGMDs)
    in pregnancy, 901
Lithium
    in headache prevention during pregnancy and lactation, 856, 860
Local anesthetics
    during labor and delivery
        seizures related to
            systemic toxicity–associated, 829–830
Lumbosacral plexus nerve injury
    birth trauma–related, 831
Lymphocytic hypophysitis
    during pregnancy
        imaging of, 812–813

M

Magnetic resonance imaging (MRI)
    during pregnancy
        of brain, 919–920
        of neurologic conditions, 795
Median neuropathy at wrist
    in pregnancy, 891
Meningitis
    during labor and delivery
        anesthesia-related, 826
Meralgia paresthetica
    in pregnancy, 891–892
Metabolic changes
    during pregnancy
        stroke related to, 915
Metabolic myopathy
    in pregnancy, 902–903
Methylsergide
    in headache prevention during pregnancy and lactation, 856, 860
Migraine
    during pregnancy
        effects of, 836–841
        investigations for, 849

Mitochondrial myopathy
    in pregnancy, 903–904
Motor neuron disease
    in pregnancy, 904–905
MRI. *See* Magnetic resonance imaging (MRI)
MS. *See* Multiple sclerosis (MS)
Multifocal motor neuropathy
    in pregnancy, 896
Multiple sclerosis (MS)
    breastfeeding by patient with, 883–884
    described, 877–878
    features of, 878–879
    labor and delivery in patient with, 881
    in pregnancy, **877–888**
        assisted reproduction techniques, 879
        case study, 877
        counseling related to, 882
        current recommendations, 884
        delivery issues, 881
        effects of, 879–881
        future directions in, 884
        imaging of, 806–808
        management of, 882–883
            DMTs in, 882
        postpartum issues, 881–882
        prognosis of, 879
        relapse management, 882
Muscle
    acquired disorders of
        in pregnancy, 896–897
    inherited disorders of
        in pregnancy, 900–903
Myasthenia gravis
    in pregnancy, 897–898
Myotonia(s)
    nondystrophic
        in pregnancy, 902
Myotonic dystrophies
    in pregnancy, 901

N

Naratriptan
    for headaches during pregnancy and lactation, 853, 858
Narcolepsy
    during pregnancy, 932–934
Neoplasm(s)
    during pregnancy
        imaging of, 809
Neurologic conditions
    in patient receiving obstetric anesthesia

Neurologic (*continued*)
    complications related to, **823–833**. *See also specific complications and* Obstetric
        anesthesia, neurologic complications in patient receiving
    during pregnancy
        imaging of, **791–822**
Neuromuscular disorders
    in pregnancy, **889–911**
        acquired disorders of muscle, 896–897
        acquired disorders of peripheral nerves, 895–896
        acquired root, plexus, and peripheral nerve lesions, 891–895
        AIDP, 895–896
        ALS, 904–905
        arthrogryposis, 899
        case study, 905–906
        Charcot-Marie-tooth disease, 899–900
        CIDP, 896
        congenital nemaline rod myopathy, 902
        described, 889–890
        disorders of neuromuscular junction, 897–899
        femoral neuropathy, 893–894
        FSHD, 900
        HBPN, 900
        HNPP, 900
        idiopathic facial nerve palsy, 894
        inflammatory muscle disease, 896–897
        inherited disorders of muscle, 900–903
        inherited disorders of peripheral nerves, 899–900
        intercostal neuralgia, 895
        lateral femoral cutaneous neuropathy, 891–892
        LGMDs, 901
        median neuropathy at wrist, 891
        metabolic myopathy, 902–903
        mitochondrial myopathy, 903–904
        motor neuron disease, 904–905
        multifocal motor neuropathy, 896
        myasthenia gravis, 897–898
        myotonic dystrophies, 901
        nonodystrophic myotonias, 902
        obturator neuropathy, 894
        periodic paralysis, 902
        postpartum foot drop
            focal peripheral nerve and root lesions–related, 892–893
        radial neuropathy, 895
        SMA, 904
        TNMG, 899
Neuromuscular junction
    disorders of
        in pregnancy, 897–899
Neuropathy(ies). *See specific types*
Nondystrophic myotonias
    in pregnancy, 902

Nonsteroidal anti-inflammatory drugs (NSAIDs)
    for headaches during pregnancy and lactation, 850, 851
NSAIDs. *See* Nonsteroidal anti-inflammatory drugs (NSAIDs)

O

Obstetric anesthesia
    neurologic complications in patient receiving, **823–833**
        anterior spinal artery syndrome, 826–827
        back pain, 829
        birth trauma, 830–831
            diagnosis and management of, 831–832
        cauda equina syndrome, 827
        direct spinal cord injury, 824
        epidural abscess, 825–826
        epidural hematoma, 825
        incidence of, 823
        meningitis, 826
        pneumocephalus, 830
        postdural puncture headache, 827–828
        seizures
            systemic toxicity of local anesthetics–related, 829–830
        total spinal block, 828–829
Obturator nerve injury
    birth trauma–related, 831
Obturator neuropathy
    in pregnancy, 894
Opiates
    for headaches during pregnancy and lactation, 852, 857

P

Pain
    back
        during labor and delivery
            anesthesia-related, 829
        during pregnancy
            imaging of, 813–816
Paradoxic embolism
    stroke due to, 919
Parasellar abnormalities
    during pregnancy
        imaging of, 809–813
Parenchymal abnormalities
    during pregnancy
        imaging of, 801–809
            AFE, 804–805
            epilepsy/seizures, 808
            gestational trophoblastic disease, 809
            MS, 806–808

Parenchymal (*continued*)
        neoplasms, 809
        postpartum angiopathy, 803–804
        preeclampsia, 801–803
        Wernicke encephalopathy, 805–806
Perinatal period
    neurologic conditions during
        imaging of, **791–822**. *See also* Pregnancy, neurologic conditions during, imaging of
Periodic paralysis
    in pregnancy, 902
Peripartum cardiomyopathy
    stroke due to, 918
Peripheral nerves
    acquired disorders of
        in pregnancy, 895–896
    inherited disorders of
        in pregnancy, 899–900
Phenytoin
    in women with epilepsy during postpartum period, 871
Pituitary abnormalities
    during pregnancy
        imaging of, 809–813
            lymphocytic hypophysitis, 812–813
            pituitary apoplexy, 809
            Sheehan syndrome, 809
            tumors, 810–812
Pituitary apoplexy
    during pregnancy
        imaging of, 809
Pituitary tumors
    during pregnancy
        imaging of, 810–812
Pneumocephalus
    during labor and delivery
        anesthesia-related, 830
Postdural puncture headache
    during labor and delivery
        anesthesia-related, 827–828
Postpartum period
    angiopathy in
        imaging of, 803–804
    focal peripheral nerve and root lesions–related foot drop in, 892–893
    headaches in, 842
    in MS patients, 881–882
    in women with epilepsy, **867–875**. *See also* Epilepsy, postpartum period in women with
Preeclampsia
    in CBF
        vs. physiologic changes in pregnancy, 782–783
    in gastroesophageal sphincter
        vs. physiologic changes in pregnancy, 784
    in hematologic changes

    vs. physiologic changes in pregnancy, 783
  during pregnancy
    imaging of, 801–803
  stroke due to, 915–916
Pregnancy
  anatomic changes during, 791–793
  brain tumors during, **937–946**. *See also* Brain tumors, during pregnancy
  cardiovascular changes during, 781–783
  drugs during
    safety of, 849
  gastrointestinal changes during, 785
  headache in, **835–866**. *See also* Headache(s), in pregnancy
  hematologic changes during, 783
  hemorrhages in
    treatment of, 922
  immunologic changes during, 784–785
  MS and, **877–888**. *See also* Multiple sclerosis (MS), in pregnancy
  neurologic conditions during
    imaging of, **791–822**. *See also* Preeclampsia; *specific disorders, e.g.,* Multiple
      sclerosis (MS)
      back pain and spinal conditions, 813–816
      contrast administration in, 795–796
      intracranial hypotension, 816
      MRI, 795
      parasellar abnormalities, 809–813
      parenchymal abnormalities, 801–809
      pituitary abnormalities, 809–813
      protocols, 793–796
      radiation exposure during, 794–795
      study selection and safety, 793–794
      vascular disorders, 796–801
  neuromuscular disorders in, **889–911**. *See also* Neuromuscular disorders,
    in pregnancy
  physiologic adaptations to, **781–789,** 792
    case study, 785–787
    clinical correlate, 785
    stroke related to
      timing of, 914–915
    vs. preeclampsia in CBF, 782–783
    vs. preeclampsia in gastroesophageal sphincter, 784
    vs. preeclampsia in hematologic changes, 783
  renal changes during, 784
  respiratory changes during, 783–784
  sleep disorders in, **925–936**. *See also* Sleep disorders, in pregnancy
  sleep during
    duration, architecture, and quality of, 925–926
  stroke in, **913–924**. *See also* Stroke, in pregnancy
  trophic effect of, 809
Puerperium
  stroke in
    risk factors for, 914

R

Radial neuropathy
  in pregnancy, 895
RCVS. *See* Reversible cerebral vasoconstriction syndrome (RCVS)
Respiratory system
  pregnancy effects on, 783–784
Restless legs syndrome
  during pregnancy, 927–930
Reversible cerebral vasoconstriction syndrome (RCVS)
  stroke due to, 916–917
Rizatriptan
  for headaches during pregnancy and lactation, 853, 858

S

Safety issues
  in women with epilepsy during postpartum period, 872–873
Seizure(s)
  during labor and delivery
    anesthesia-related
      systemic toxicity of local anesthetics, 829–830
  during pregnancy
    imaging of, 808
Selective serotonin reuptake inhibitors (SSRIs)
  in headache prevention during pregnancy and lactation, 855, 859
Sheehan syndrome
  during pregnancy
    imaging of, 809
Sleep
  in pregnancy
    duration, architecture, and quality of, 925–926
Sleep-disordered breathing
  during pregnancy, 930–932
Sleep disorders
  in pregnancy, **925–936**
    hypersomnia, 932–934
    insomnia, 926–927
    narcolepsy, 932–934
    restless legs syndrome, 927–930
    sleep-disordered breathing, 930–932
SMA. *See* Spinal muscular atrophy (SMA)
Spinal conditions
  during pregnancy
    imaging of, 813–816
Spinal cord injury
  direct
    during labor and delivery
      anesthesia-related, 824
Spinal muscular atrophy (SMA)
  in pregnancy, 904

SSRIs. *See* Selective serotonin reuptake inhibitors (SSRIs)
Stroke
   in pregnancy, **913–924**
      causes of, 915–919
         AFE, 918–919
         choriocarcinoma, 918
         CVST, 917–918
         eclampsia, 915–916
         general, 919
         paradoxic embolism, 919
         peripartum cardiomyopathy, 918
         preeclampsia, 915–916
         RCVS, 916–917
      diagnosis of
         imaging in, 797–801, 919–920
      prevalence of, 913
      prevention of, 920–921
      risk factors for, 914
      timing of, 914–915
      treatment of, 921–922
Subarachnoid hemorrhage
   during pregnancy
      imaging of, 796
Sumatriptan
   for headaches during pregnancy and lactation, 853, 857–858

T

TCAs. *See* Tricyclic antidepressants (TCAs)
Tension-type headache
   during pregnancy
      effects of, 836
      investigations for, 848–849
Thrombolytic therapy
   in pregnancy-related stroke management, 921
Thrombosis(es)
   cerebral venous and sinus
      stroke due to, 917–918
   venous
      during pregnancy
         imaging of, 797–801
TNMG. *See* Transient neonatal myasthenia gravis (TNMG)
Topiramate
   in headache prevention during pregnancy and lactation, 855, 860
   in women with epilepsy during postpartum period, 872
Total spinal block
   during labor and delivery
      anesthesia-related, 828–829
Transient neonatal myasthenia gravis (TNMG)
   in pregnancy, 899

Trauma
    obstetric birth–related
        anesthesia-related, 830–831
        neuropathy due to
            diagnosis and management of, 831–832
Tricyclic antidepressants (TCAs)
    in headache prevention during pregnancy and lactation, 854, 859
Triptans
    for headaches during pregnancy and lactation, 853, 857–858
Tumor(s)
    brain
        during pregnancy, **937–946**. See also Brain tumors, during pregnancy
    pituitary
        during pregnancy
            imaging of, 810–812

V

Valproic acid
    in headache prevention during pregnancy and lactation, 856, 860
    in women with epilepsy during postpartum period, 871
Vascular disorders
    during pregnancy
        headache and, 843–846
        imaging of, 796–801
            stroke, 797–801
            subarachnoid hemorrhage, 796
            venous thrombosis, 797–801
Venous thrombosis
    during pregnancy
        imaging of, 797–801

W

Wernicke encephalopathy
    during pregnancy
        imaging of, 805–806
Wrist
    median neuropathy at
        in pregnancy, 891

Z

Zonisamide
    in women with epilepsy during postpartum period, 872

Moving?

Make sure your subscription moves with you!

To notify us of your new address, find your **Clinics Account Number** (located on your mailing label above your name), and contact customer service at:

Email: journalscustomerservice-usa@elsevier.com

800-654-2452 (subscribers in the U.S. & Canada)
314-447-8871 (subscribers outside of the U.S. & Canada)

Fax number: 314-447-8029

Elsevier Health Sciences Division
Subscription Customer Service
3251 Riverport Lane
Maryland Heights, MO 63043

*To ensure uninterrupted delivery of your subscription, please notify us at least 4 weeks in advance of move.

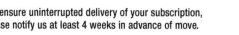